Kristine Napier, M.P.H., R.D., L.D.

EAT AWAY
DIABETES

Beat Type 2 Diabetes by Winning the Blood-Sugar Battle

Prentice Hall Press
a member of Penguin Putnam Inc.
New York

This publication contains the opinions and ideas of its author and is designed to provide use-ful advice in regard to the subject matter covered. The author and publisher are not engaged in rendering medical or other professional services in this publication. This publication is not intended to provide a basis for action in particular circumstances without consideration by a competent health professional. The author and publisher expressly disclaim any responsibility for any liability, loss, or risk, personal or otherwise, which is incurred as a consequence, directly or indirectly, of the use and application of any of the contents of this book.

a member of Penguin Putnam Inc.
375 Hudson Street
New York, New York 10014

www.penguinputnam.com

Copyright © 2002 by Kristine Napier

Prentice Hall® is a registered trademark of Pearson Education, Inc.
All rights reserved. No part of this book may be reproduced in any form or by any means, without permission in writing from the publisher. Published simultaneously in Canada

Acquisitions Editor: *Ed Claflin*
Production Editor: *Sharon L. Gonzalez*
Page Design/Layout: *Robyn Beckerman*

Library of Congress Cataloging-in-Publication Data

Napier, Kristine M.
    Eat away diabetes / Kristine Napier.
        p.   cm.
    Includes index.
    ISBN 0-13-032042-0—ISBN 0-7352-0251-6 (pbk.)
    1. Non-insulin-dependent diabetes—Diet therapy.   2. Non-insulin-dependent diabetes—Diet therapy—Recipes.   I. Title.

    RC662 .N344   2002
    616.4'620654—dc21   2002022020

Printed in the United States of America

10   9   8   7   6   5   4   3   2

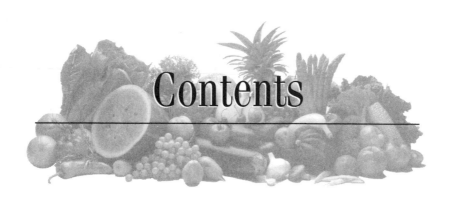

Contents

Contents

Acknowledgments

Translating the science of living well with Type 2 diabetes into everyday actions is not easy. I extend a heartfelt thank you to the people who have made this process easier—and who have therefore contributed substantially to this book: Dr. Byron Hoogwerf, Dr. Joanne Findlay, Dr. Jerry Goldstone, Dr. Fred Pashkow, and to my nutrition colleague, Melissa Stevens. For his exuberant enthusiasm in shaping this book and corralling my thoughts, a resounding thank you to Ed the editor (Ed Claflin). A most humble thank you to my culinary assistants Nancy Morgan (my indispensable culinary manager), Sara Stuhan, Sarah Wilson, Molly McPolin, Sarah Kosknosky, and Kristy Simmelink, whose hard work, long hours, and stained aprons played a most important role in creating the recipes in this book. Last and certainly not least: my love and thanks to my husband, Jim, and my children Susie and Jimmy for supporting me through this endeavor.

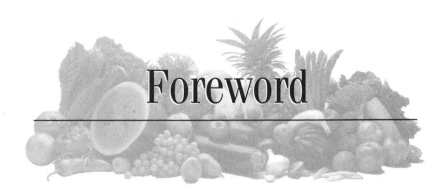

Foreword

Several years ago, the American Diabetes Association initiated the slogan "Diabetes is serious."

To the people who deal with the consequences of diabetes every day—including millions of patients, members of their families, and their health care team—this statement rings true. In fact, I believe that many of the health care workers who have witnessed the complications of this disease would join me in saying that diabetes is one of the *most* serious diseases that we are dealing with today.

Despite improving therapies for treating diabetes, and strategies for preventing its onset, the number of people with Type 2 diabetes continues to increase to the point where it will soon be a global epidemic. Today, in the United States, there are more than sixteen million people who have diabetes. Diabetes is the leading cause of blindness, the need for dialysis, and nontraumatic leg amputations; diabetes more than doubles the risks for heart attacks and strokes.

These statistics are staggering. But Kristine Napier, in this wonderfully useful book, is not dealing with statistics. Here, she has advice for each individual, including you.

If you already have Type 2 diabetes, Kris gives you the guidelines to help reduce the risk for complications. More specifically, she gives you the nutritional help that can help you gain control over the disease.

If you do not have diabetes, you are probably aware of the factors associated with future risk for diabetes. Are you overweight or sedentary? These are just two factors. Many other factors come into play, including your genetic makeup. But there is a good chance you can exercise control over these factors if you follow the dietary and nutritional guidelines that are advocated by Kris and described in this book.

Kris's advice is all the more sound and practical because she has had diabetes herself. Through hard-won experience, she has discovered that the best diet is the kind that's made up of delicious food and tempting recipes.

Each one of the scores of recipes in this book was developed by Kris to help keep her own diabetes under control. She discovered that she could make meals that the whole family would relish—yes, even a picky teenager! In the process of developing these recipes, she made the "food discoveries" that would improve the health of each person in her family.

Kris also knows how to talk about diabetes so that people can understand. That is a notable ability. Whether she is recounting important findings about the nutritional habits of the Pima Indians, or describing the role of LDL-c receptors, the pictures created by her words are clear and precise. (Think of those receptors as "grappling hooks," she suggests! Think of poor nutrition as a way of "burning the fine furniture" in your house!)

In addition, Kris creates a clear link between the authoritative guidelines developed by research specialists and the practical concerns of people who want day-to-day advice in guarding their personal health. In previewing this book, I was struck by how well her advice conforms to the guidelines recommended by such standard-setting organizations as the American Diabetes Association (ADA) and the American Heart Association (AHA). Napier excels in bringing those recommendations within reach of every reader. Her practical suggestions, her easy tips for lifestyle modification, and above all, her skill as a cook as well as nutritionist make the ADA and AHA advice far easier to understand. The result is a book that's more than a source of information—it is a source of advice and guidelines that deserves a prominent place on every kitchen shelf.

Lifestyle change, as Napier points out, does require some effort. But she herself is living proof that the practical implementation of her methods has a real payoff. I only hope that every reader, after seeing this book, will feel convinced and motivated to implement the lifestyle changes that Napier recommends. You *can* control Type 2 diabetes—that's essential good news for the millions of people with diabetes. For the millions more who want to reduce the risk for diabetes, this book is an indispensable guide, your best hope yet—a chance at prevention.

Byron J. Hoogwerf, M.D., F.A.C.P., C.D.E., F.A.C.E.
Cleveland Clinic Foundation
Cleveland, OH

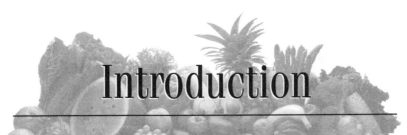

Introduction

Type 2 Diabetes: An American Epidemic . . . with a Solution

Why is Type 2 diabetes now such an urgent concern? Why do diabetes experts now recommend that the 15.7 million Americans with Type 2 diabetes undergo *more* aggressive treatment for *lower* blood sugars? Why are we so worried about the growing number of people with undiagnosed Type 2 diabetes? And why do we fret about people who don't even have diabetes but who have a condition called glucose intolerance?

Worse yet, why are we now concerned about people with Type 2 diabetes who are taking medications or are on insulin to control their blood sugars, and who supposedly have good blood sugar control? Believe it or not, some diabetes medications actually cause many diabetics to gain weight, which worsens their blood sugar levels and increases their need for medications—and creates a vicious cycle. Indeed, diabetes medications are a double-edged sword, and sometimes the undesired edge cuts deeper than the desired one.

And why is it up to you to fight a myth believed by so many physicians who care for people with Type 2 diabetes? British diabetes expert Gareth Williams, M.D., writes in the *International Journal of Obesity,* "There is a commonly held myth amongst physicians that Type 2 diabetes is a relatively mild disease which is easily managed." It is up to you to tell your physician that you want to take charge of treating your diabetes more aggressively and to bring it under strict control.

Reasons to Worry About Type 2 Diabetes

If you have Type 2 diabetes, you have more to worry about than a number (your blood sugar reading, that is) that falls off the precipice of high normal.

Today, the complications of Type 2 diabetes make it the seventh leading cause of death in America. That is why it's called the "silent killer." Heaped on top of the fact that many people with Type 2 diabetes aren't properly treated—"controlled," in diabetes-speak—one-third of Type 2 diabetics don't know that their blood sugar levels are ranging out of control. Many people with undiagnosed Type 2 diabetes don't know they have it until some associated serious health problem crops up. The first warning of diabetes in many people, for example, is a heart attack or stroke.

Indeed, undiagnosed diabetes, as well as diagnosed diabetes that is not controlled properly, can wreak serious damage on one or more body systems. Here are some of the alarming and frightening complications and associated statistics:

- Blindness or other eye complications: Diabetes is the leading cause of new cases of blindness in people ages 20 to 74. Each year 12,000 to 24,000 people lose their sight because of diabetes.

- Kidney damage: Diabetes is the leading cause of end-stage kidney disease, a condition where a person requires dialysis or a kidney transplant to live. Ten to twenty-one percent of all people with diabetes will develop kidney disease.

- Nerve damage, infections, and amputations: A person with diabetes is fifteen to forty times more likely to have an amputation of a toe, foot, or leg than is someone without diabetes. Each year more than fifty-six thousand diabetics must have an amputation.

- Heart disease and stroke: People with diabetes are two to four times more likely to have atherosclerotic, or artery-clogging, heart disease. Heart disease, in fact, is a contributing factor to three-quarters of diabetes-related deaths. Diabetes causes stroke risk to skyrocket, *at least* doubling and possibly quadrupling it.

Before you say, "Those are just statistics," I'm going to give you a glimpse at a group of people with diabetes as a reality check on the potential complications of having diabetes. Diabetes experts at Emory University School of Medicine in Atlanta, Georgia, scrutinized 121 of their Type 2 diabetic patients. This group had an average age of 63 and had been diagnosed with Type 2 diabetes for an average of twelve years. Here is what they found:

- 80 percent had high blood pressure (hypertension)
- 78 percent had nerve damage (neuropathy)
- 64 percent (about two-thirds) had abnormally high blood cholesterol readings (hyperlipidemia)
- 22 percent had eye damage (retinopathy)
- 21 percent had kidney abnormalities (albuminuria, or protein in the urine)

More Cause for Concern: An Epidemic on the Rise

The urgent concern over diabetes isn't just as a result of medical experts knowing more about the dangers of Type 2 diabetes and the critical importance of more exacting control of blood sugars. Alarm bells sound repeatedly now at the virtual epidemic of Type 2 diabetes, given its tenfold increase from 1982 to 1994. An estimated 15.7 million Americans now have Type 2 diabetes. Worse yet, the warning bells sound at younger and younger ages. At one time Type 2 diabetes was virtually unheard of until the fourth decade of life. It was only in 1979 that doctors first diagnosed it in teenagers (the first diagnoses came in Native American teenagers, who are predisposed to being overweight).

Pediatric Annals, published by pediatric diabetes experts from Children's Hospital at the University of Pittsburgh, recently reported that this diabetes epidemic is worldwide. In 1995 there were an estimated 135 million Type 2 diabetics in the world. That number is expected to more than double by 2025—to 300 million.

Why are so many more people developing Type 2 diabetes, especially at younger ages, and why has this disease now invaded even the lives of children? The incidence is increasing rapidly because so many more Americans are overweight, obese, and/or sedentary. The latest health statistics tell us that at least one-third of Americans are obese and that 58 percent are overweight. Indeed, the fact that young people are tending to exceed a healthy weight explains why more and more kids are getting this adult disease.

Remember that group of people studied by Emory University School of Medicine? Another striking statistic about this group was that their average body mass index (BMI) was 31. A body mass index over 25 indicates a person is overweight, and those with a BMI over 28 have a greatly increased chance of developing Type 2 diabetes. As you will soon learn, most of these people wouldn't have any evidence of Type 2 diabetes if they brought their weight down and adopted an overall healthier lifestyle.

It is not just Americans who are getting heavier. People in countries all over the world are carrying more and more excess weight. The prevalence of obesity in established market economies in Europe, Canada, and Australia is rising rapidly. In what has come as a great surprise to world health experts, obesity rates are rising even in Asia, which is showing one of the sharpest increases in Type 2 diabetes.

Now for the Good News

Believe it or not, here is where the good news comes in:

Eating more healthfully and the cascade of wonderful health advantages that result can virtually wipe out Type 2 diabetes.

That's right: Losing excess weight, adopting a specific eating style, and exercising regularly can drop sugar levels back down to normal levels. There is a huge advantage to normalizing blood sugars. It assists in warding off complications such as blindness, heart disease, infections, and amputations. We are not just guessing that this helps. There is solid proof that intensive therapy which controls blood sugars will prevent the microvascular complications (damage to blood vessels in the eyes, kidneys, and heart, etc., as noted above) of Type 2 diabetes.

You simply have to take control—take charge—of your health destiny.

Granted, achieving better control isn't easy. It is downright difficult. Making the necessary lifestyle changes is so difficult that many diabetes experts throw up their hands in desperation and say they can do no better than hold the current ground. But don't give up on yourself. You can help yourself. You can make your diabetes disappear.

What This Book Will Do for You

I am going to teach you how to eat your way out of diabetes—permanently. This book will walk you (literally as well as figuratively) through a complete understanding of this potentially killer disease and empower you to take action; it will give you the knowledge needed to do so.

You will learn the new diagnostic and treatment guidelines, and understand why it is so important to jump into action at the first indication that your sugar levels are starting to rise. What is more, I will describe the latest news from the American Diabetes Association, which favors treatment at much lower levels of elevated fasting blood sugars than it did just a few years ago, but also when fasting levels are normal but blood sugar levels are high two hours after eating a meal.

This book will eliminate any confusion about how important it is to treat Type 2 diabetes. You will no longer be one of those who have been led to believe that "a little bit of extra blood sugar" isn't bad for them. You will be empowered by knowing that all diabetics—even those with a little bit of high blood sugar—should be treated aggressively.

I'm also going to clarify every confusing detail about eating carbohydrates when you have Type 2 diabetes. You may have heard two very disparate facts about carbohydrates—that you should be following a high-protein, low-carbohydrate diet and that some diabetes experts say diabetics can have simple carbohydrates such as candy and soda pop as long as they count their numbers. Read on to learn the truth.

You may also be wondering about the potential help and also the possible dangers of certain dietary supplements that have been recommended for diabetics, such as chromium and stevia. You'll learn here what you need to know.

Most important, all this science and advice will be converted into dinner table strategies, into food that you can put on your plate to achieve the best possible health. Yes, you will find recipes suitable for diabetics at every stage of getting their disease under control as well as menus at many calorie levels that you can use every day.

I Know You Can Do It Because I Did

No matter how heavy you are now and no matter how much out of control your blood sugars are today, you can lose the weight and control your sugars. Let me tell you my story.

I was a long-distance racer and a young dietitian who did not understand how people could let themselves get heavy and suffer the resultant health consequences (such as becoming a diabetic). But then I suffered a series of health troubles that resulted in my own blossoming weight—and Type 2 diabetes. In my late twenties I was diagnosed with systemic lupus. For a long time, despite high corticosteroid doses (a drug that often leads to weight gain), I managed to control my weight. But then my disease worsened, and I became increasingly disabled physically. Long gone were my running days; I was lucky to get up out of a chair to care for my children. By my late thirties I was seriously overweight and still required corticosteroid medications to control the lupus. That is when the doctor told me I had Type 2 diabetes.

Granted, my diabetes was spurred by the medication (which not only causes weight gain but also causes Type 2 diabetes even in people who are not overweight) more than it was by my being overweight. But I was truly in a bind. How could I get the weight down when I couldn't move very much and was still on the weight-gain drug? By this time I was in a wheelchair because the disease had eaten away both hips.

It was a long haul for me to get the weight off and bring my sugars down. I had many seemingly impossible battles to fight, but I did it. I never thought that I would see a day without three or four shots of insulin, but here I am, still on the corticosteroid medicine, slightly hobbled, but managing to find a way to stay in shape and avoid the complications of Type 2 diabetes.

The point of telling you this is to give you hope that no matter how hopeless your situation seems, I'll help you find a way to exercise and lose those pounds that are making you diabetic. We'll do it together.

Understanding = Empowerment

I am a firm believer in empowerment through knowledge. If you have Type 2 diabetes, you need to know exactly why you have this condition. You also need to know what effect it has on your metabolism and on every system in your body (especially your heart). To bring you to this understanding, I'll first walk you through your lifestyle factors and help you see that what you do during the course of your daily life contributes to having Type 2 diabetes or making it worse. Then we'll look into your pancreas, liver, and cells to show you what is happening to them because you have this disease.

As we help you pick apart the food you eat, you will understand how food impacts your metabolism, your blood sugars, and therefore your health. Then you'll learn how to put together the right foods in the form of great recipes you can use every day to eat your way out of Type 2 diabetes. You'll understand how food can help you get better and avoid the complications associated with diabetes.

This understanding equals empowerment.

And empowerment enables you to spring into action and take the steps you need to eliminate this disease from your life (or, at the very least, control it to eliminate complications). So grab a highlighting marker and some sticky notes, and start reading. You will need to concentrate, so find a good place to study.

Chapter One

All About Type 2 Diabetes

What's in a Name?

If you are confused about the name of Type 2 diabetes mellitus, you are not alone. Let's start with the basic terms of *diabetes* and *mellitus*. Many times Type 2 diabetes mellitus is shortened to Type 2 diabetes. *Diabetes* is a Latin word with several meanings, one of which is to "siphon off," and *mellitus* is from the Greek for "honey-sweet." That is exactly what happens when you have either Type 1 or Type 2 diabetes: the body siphons off sugar from the bloodstream through the kidneys (they act as the siphon) and out through the urine. That is why so many people say, "I have sugar," when they learn they have diabetes. Indeed, we all have sugar in our bloodstream (we need it for energy). In diabetes mellitus the body doesn't know how to handle the sugar properly, so it works hard to get rid of it. This process of figuring out that there is too much sugar (glucose) and then getting rid of it is very hard on the body—which is what causes complications.

(Note: Type 1 diabetes mellitus has a very different cause and treatment that is not covered in this book. "Diabetes" in this book refers to Type 2 diabetes mellitus.)

Over the years Type 2 diabetes has had a couple of names, including adult-onset diabetes mellitus (AODM) and non-insulin-dependent diabetes mellitus (NIDDM). Both of these are indeed confusing, and neither is correct.

Adult-onset diabetes no longer accurately describes the age of onset. As you read in the Introduction, the age at which people develop this type of diabetes is dropping steadily. Today, teens and even children are afflicted with this formerly adult-only disease because of the alarming epidemic of obesity. So the name adult-onset diabetes is not appropriate.

The name non-insulin-dependent diabetes mellitus is also confusing and seemingly inaccurate to nonmedical people, especially those with Type 2 diabetes who need injectable insulin. The term was originally coined to distinguish Type 2 from what is now called Type I, which had been called insulin-dependent diabetes. Before continuing to explain these terms and why both are outdated, I would like to take a detour to explain insulin.

More Facts About Insulin That You Need to Know

Insulin is a hormone produced by the pancreas to help the body use glucose. After you eat, food is broken down into its most basic parts—amino acids (from the protein in your food), fatty acids (from the fat in your food), and glucose (from the carbohydrate in your food)—and then absorbed into the bloodstream. Glucose is what affects the pancreas and how much insulin it sends out.

Glucose is the body's main source of fuel; in fact, it is the best source of fuel. But glucose in the bloodstream is useless to the body (and, as you will see, becomes a villain) unless it can enter the cells and be burned. Think of it this way: Your car needs fuel to run, which is gasoline. You can fill up your tank with gas, but unless the gas leaves the tank and enters the engine, the car will not run even if you have a full tank. So it is with glucose. Unless it leaves the bloodstream, your cells cannot use it as fuel.

Here is where insulin comes in. When the body's metabolic machinery is working properly, the pancreas senses this surge of glucose and says, "Time to start pumping out insulin." Put another way, insulin is the key that unlocks the door of each cell to allow glucose to enter. There it can be burned. This is good for two reasons: First, you get the fuel you need to live, work, and play. Second, your blood glucose levels don't rise too high.

In Type 2 diabetes the body's metabolic machinery does not work properly, so although insulin is pumped out, the body is "insulin resistant." This means the body resists the action of insulin. A person with Type 2 diabetes produces insulin, but the insulin won't unlock the cell door anymore—at least with normal amounts of insulin. The body then starts producing lots and lots of insulin, and finally all those keys let the glucose into the cells. Blood glucose levels eventually return to normal, but there are disastrous consequences, which will be discussed later in this chapter.

Many Type 2 diabetics never need injected insulin, while others do. In fact, because more and more people are getting heavier and heavier, and as a result are developing Type 2 diabetes—and more severe cases—more people need injected insulin.

Those with Type I diabetes, formerly called insulin-dependent diabetes mellitus, always need some form of insulin therapy, such as injected insulin or an insulin pump. Since their pancreas cannot produce insulin, they would quickly die without insulin therapy.

Let me quickly add here that if you have Type 2 diabetes and currently take insulin injections, do not stop taking them. You may be very sick without it, risking a coma or even death. It is my hope to empower you to change your lifestyle, lose weight, exercise, and reach the point when your need for insulin injections is nothing or next to nothing. Please keep in mind that all this change must be supervised by your doctor.

As we have seen, the term *non-insulin dependent diabetes mellitus* is inappropriate, which is why the American Diabetes Association recommends that we use *Type 2 diabetes*.

Why You Got This Disease

So what is it? Genetics, family history, what you ate for dinner the night before you were diagnosed with diabetes? What exactly caused you to come down with this disease that seems to be turning your life upside down and demanding that you make some lifestyle changes? For the most part your current lifestyle has led you, probably gradually, to what we know is the serious metabolic disorder of Type 2 diabetes, which at one time people said was "just a little bit of high blood sugar."

Risk Factors for Type 2 Diabetes

Category 1: Risk Factors You Cannot Eliminate but You Can Influence

- Genetics (family history)
- Race
- In utero (inside your mother's womb) conditions
- Increasing age

Category 2: Risk Factors You Can Eliminate

- Excess weight
- Excess weight around your middle
- Couch potato syndrome—being too sedentary
- Eating a diet too high in fat, especially saturated fat

Most likely one or all of the following three factors have placed you at increased risk of getting Type 2 diabetes:

1. You may have a genetic predisposition or family tendency.
2. Race: People of certain races, including Hispanics (especially from Mexico and Latin America), African Americans, and Native Americans (especially the Pimas). According to the National Institutes of Health, Native Americans, Hispanics, and other non-white peoples have up to ten times the rate of diabetes as Caucasians.
3. How your mother ate while pregnant with you and how much weight she gained. (See the sidebar regarding the exciting new field of research on fetal programming.)

If you have one or more of these factors working against you, does that mean your fate is sealed and that you will get Type 2 diabetes?

Absolutely not.

We call these factors that are always and forever in the underlying makeup of your cells *risk factors,* but I like to use another term: *influence-*

able risk factors. While you cannot erase or eliminate these factors from the makeup of your cells, you can influence their expression.

Let me draw an analogy before going into more detail.

The Chinese had an ancient custom of binding a young girl's feet so they would not grow. If a girl had the genetic predisposition to a size 9 foot, the act of binding her feet from a young age kept this genetic tendency from expressing itself. The same is true of Type 2 diabetes. By taking certain actions (which you will learn so that they become second nature), you can keep the tendency of Type 2 diabetes from expressing itself.

How You Can Change Your Influenceable Risk Factors

In most cases the influence of genetics, race, or in utero conditions expresses itself only if you become too heavy or too sedentary—or, worse yet, too heavy and too sedentary. You will develop Type 2 diabetes if you have these factors in the background by hanging on to those extra pounds and your worn-out spot on the couch (from sitting there too much!).

Indeed, research has taught us that Type 2 diabetes is the result of environment, or lifestyle, plus these unchangeable factors. This means that you can prevent or at least delay its onset. In medicine we learn a great deal about certain diseases by studying those who tend to get them more often than usual (this is called epidemiology). Studying Type 2 diabetes in the Pima Indians has taught us that lifestyle is just as important as genes. Today, one out of every two Pima Indians is struck by diabetes at an incredibly early age. This has only happened since their lifestyle has changed. National Institutes of Health (NIH) researchers have studied at least 90 percent of those on the reservation where they live.

The Pima Indian Story

About thirty thousand years ago the Pima Indians were among the first people to walk the soil of the Americas. Archaeologists think that they descended from a prehistoric people who originated in Mexico. In the earlier years of their existence, their lives centered on hard physical work.

Fetal Programming

Recent research suggests that how your mother ate and how much weight she gained when carrying you, as well as your birth weight, influence your risk of Type 2 diabetes. From a whole new field of research called fetal programming we have learned that those born to mothers who did not gain enough weight (you read correctly) during pregnancy and were born at a smaller than average birth weight are more likely to get Type 2 diabetes later in life. In addition, offspring of mothers who were diabetic during pregnancy (called gestational diabetes)—especially if the diabetes was not controlled properly—are more likely to get Type 2 diabetes as adults.

Undernutrition. Fetal programming experts believe that suboptimal conditions in the womb—too few calories—increase the risk of adult-onset diabetes. Studies have shown that people born smaller than expected have less lean muscle mass. This tends to be the result of decreased nutrition in the middle months of pregnancy, the prime time for muscle bulk to develop.

Another reason that too few calories during gestation may increase the risk for diabetes has to do with the fetus's survival response. When calories are scarce, the developing baby learns to decrease its dependence on glucose for the energy it needs to grow.

Some two thousand years ago many moved from Mexico to the Sonoron Desert where the Gila River meets the Salt River in what is now southern Arizona. Remarkable farmers and engineers, they built a fabulous system of irrigation in this desert country and brought the countryside alive with vibrantly colored crops—wheat, beans, squash, and cotton among them. They were master weavers and turned the threads of their crop into watertight baskets.

Instead, the baby turns to secondary fuels, including amino acids, the building blocks of protein that are always floating around in the bloodstream. When conditions are very sparse, the developing baby may also break down the muscle tissue it has already built up for energy.

The problem with turning to secondary energy sources is that the cells get "rusty" at shuttling glucose into the cells. Babies growing in conditions of too few calories may permanently lose some of their ability to transfer glucose from the bloodstream into cells.

Gestational diabetes. We have learned about the possible ill effects of gestational diabetes (especially not well controlled) on the future health of the child from the Pima Indians, a group with an exceptionally high rate of Type 2 diabetes. Babies exposed in utero to high levels of blood glucose not only have more problems at birth but are also at increased risk of becoming obese and getting diabetes—and at a much earlier age. Fetal programming researchers believe this risk is in addition to any genetically increased risk they may inherit. This occurs because these babies often suffer irreparable damages to the cells in the pancreas that produce insulin. This is less likely to happen, however, if a woman with gestational diabetes keeps it under control.

The other important point central to their lives years ago—and, as it turns out, a key factor in their developing Type 2 diabetes at a young age— was their cyclical food supply for thousands of years. Like many other farming, hunting, and fishing people, the Pimas years ago experienced alternating periods of feast and famine. As geneticist James Neel first proposed in 1962, they had no choice but to adapt genetically to survive such extreme changes in caloric intake. This adaptation, called the "thrifty gene" theory, is now accepted as one of the reasons that the Pimas have such a problem with Type 2 diabetes.

Developing a thrifty gene allowed the Pimas to store fat very efficiently during the times when food was plentiful. This ability to store fat efficiently prevented them from starving when food was scarce.

Today, the Pima Indians live in the Gila River Indian Community in southern Arizona. They were forced to abandon their traditional lifestyle about one hundred years ago when their water supply was diverted by American farmers settling upstream. This was disastrous for them. Now in a desert without water, their two-thousand-year-old tradition of irrigation and agriculture abruptly came to a halt. They were struck by poverty, followed by malnutrition that led to starvation. The American government sent the Pima Indians lard, sugar, and white flour so they wouldn't starve to death. While it saved their lives, this food was significantly different from what they had been accustomed to eating for thousands of years. Let's take a look at what medical anthropologists at the NIH discovered via their intensive research.

In the 1890s the traditional Pima Indian diet consisted of only about 15 percent fat and was high in starch and fiber. Today, their diet mimics the typical Western diet and consists of almost 40 percent fat calories as well as lots of simple sugars and refined starches. Their current diet combined with their genetic adaptation of storing fat efficiently has been bad for their health. The Pimas are prone to both obesity and Type 2 diabetes. In fact, an astonishing 50 percent have the disease. Nearly all—95 percent—of those with Type 2 diabetes are overweight. They also get the disease much younger: on average, just 36 years old, compared to Caucasians who get it at about age 60 (although that age is dropping rapidly because of the dramatic rise in obesity).

Having Type 2 diabetes so much longer is extremely problematical: The longer a person has it, the greater the risk for developing complications such as kidney disease, heart disease, and eye problems leading to blindness. These diabetic complications are the leading causes of illness and death among the Pima Indians along with nerve disease that leads to infections and amputations.

Here is something else that is very telling about the critical importance of lifestyle in people at high risk for Type 2 diabetes. The NIH researchers recently visited a group of Pima Indians living as their ancestors did in a remote area of the Sierra Madre Mountains of Mexico. Genetic testing proved that this group is genetically the same as the Pimas now living in Arizona. However, only about 8 percent of them had Type 2 diabetes, and very few were overweight.

The next question is: Can a change in diet help the Pima Indians—and anyone else predisposed to Type 2 diabetes?

Yes!

The NIH researchers have determined that eating healthier—such as cutting the fat in the diet and eating higher fiber foods—as well as exercising more can prevent Type 2 diabetes from developing in the Pima Indians. This good news applies to everyone with an increased risk.

In the chapters that follow you will learn exactly how to do all these things.

The Steps That Lead to Type 2 Diabetes

Type 2 diabetes doesn't happen overnight but occurs silently in steps over five to seven years. It comes on gradually, preceded by metabolic abnormalities called insulin resistance and then impaired glucose tolerance. Let's take a closer look at these steps.

Step 1: Insulin Resistance

The first thing that happens in people who eventually are diagnosed with frank Type 2 diabetes is that they have higher than normal levels of circulating insulin because the cells are insulin-resistant. At this point the beta cells of the pancreas still sense the rise in blood glucose levels and try to compensate by producing more insulin. However, the body cells don't respond to the insulin key that is supposed to unlock the door to let the glucose in. Still trying to compensate to move the glucose from the bloodstream into the cells where it can be used for energy, the pancreas pumps out more and more insulin. In the earliest phases, some people with this abnormality can still keep blood glucose levels normal by pumping out more insulin. People who are overweight and/or physically inactive have a greater tendency toward insulin resistance.

Even though people with insulin resistance manage to maintain normal blood glucose levels, they pay a high cost. The body does not like all that circulating insulin. Here is a summary of what happens silently inside the body when insulin levels are higher than normal (even when blood glucose levels are normal):

- Triglyceride levels rise. Although research has not yet drawn a direct line between high triglyceride levels and atherosclerotic, or artery-clogging, heart disease, we do know that people with high triglycerides are at increased risk for atherosclerosis.

- HDL cholesterol (high-density lipoprotein) or good cholesterol drops. We know that the higher the HDL cholesterol levels, the lower the risk of atherosclerotic heart disease.

- The body retains sodium. Remember that old adage, "For every action, there is a reaction"? Well, the same is true with high insulin levels. One of the many things they cause is sodium retention, which can raise blood pressure.

- Blood pressure rises independent of sodium intake. In other words, blood pressure seems to go up for reasons other than sodium retention.

- Fibrinogen, or one of the blood-clotting factors, goes into overdrive. Among other things, this can lead to tiny blood clots that can clog arteries and contribute to atherosclerosis.

- LDL cholesterol (low-density lipoprotein cholesterol) or bad cholesterol particles become abnormally dense. This also increases the risk of atherosclerosis.

Insulin resistance can be present for many years before the second step toward Type 2 diabetes occurs: impaired glucose tolerance.

Step 2: Impaired Glucose Tolerance

Over time, people with insulin resistance secrete more and more insulin to move the same amount of glucose into cells where it is needed for energy. However, this ability to compensate gradually breaks down and blood glucose levels inch their way up. In other words, the beta cells of the pancreas that produce insulin still sense the increased glucose levels, but the high amounts of insulin cannot move all the glucose out of the bloodstream. Such people are said to have impaired glucose tolerance. Many people remain undiagnosed at this point, but damage is already occurring in many organs and blood vessels.

Step 3: Full-Blown Type 2 Diabetes

In full-blown Type 2 diabetes the beta cells in the pancreas cannot produce enough insulin, and blood glucose levels climb even higher.

There is another reason that the blood glucose levels rise. When the beta cells still sense high blood glucose levels and produce insulin, the body sensors get the message that there is enough energy available to live. However, when insulin production is less than optimal, the body says, "Hey, we're short on energy." Trying to help solve the energy crisis, the liver responds by giving up its stores of glucose. This only makes matters worse by raising blood glucose levels even more.

How Excess Body Weight Brings on Type 2 Diabetes

According to statistics from the National Institutes of Health in September 2000, about 80 to 90 percent of people with Type 2 diabetes are also overweight. So what comes first? Overweight or insulin resistance? The most prominent theories say that obesity comes first and causes insulin resistance.

Here is the evidence for this line of thinking: We know for certain that fatty (adipose) tissue produces a number of substances that probably interfere with the body's usual ability to control glucose levels. Some of these substances pumped out by fatty tissue include the following:

- Non-esterified fatty acids: These may be especially important in causing insulin resistance. They may do so by interfering with the movement of glucose in the cells; stimulating too much insulin secretion; causing the liver to produce too much glucose; and/or increasing the amount of triglycerides in tissues other than fatty tissue.
- Tumor necrosis factor alpha, which may inhibit normal insulin activity.
- A hormone called leptin.

Other theories suggest that obesity and insulin resistance are not related to each other but arise from some common or totally distinct (or uncommon) processes.

Whichever is the case, the most important message is that weight reduction improves insulin sensitivity. There is no question about that.

Using certain medications to improve insulin sensitivity generally does not help people lose weight. On the contrary, such treatments often cause weight gain.

Why Couch Potatoes Are More at Risk for Type 2 Diabetes

The human body was meant to move, to be active every day. We were built to maintain a certain amount of strong muscle tissue.

Inactivity has disastrous consequences on the human body, especially when it comes to insulin sensitivity. Simply put, people who stay active and keep their muscles working are more likely to have cells that are appropriately sensitive to the effects of insulin. They are less likely to develop insulin resistance that can develop into Type 2 diabetes.

Here are some of the important research findings that prove this:

- Exercise increases blood flow to the muscles, which also increases the ability of the blood to transport certain substances.

- Exercise and increased blood flow boosts the ability of muscle tissue to metabolize substances.

- Exercise helps cells take up glucose and dispose of it more rapidly—independent of the need for insulin. This insulin-independent uptake of glucose into the muscle cells is thought to last for about two hours after exercise.

- After exercise, in what is called the recovery period, glucose is shuttled to muscle tissue more rapidly. This not only helps muscles store glucose as glycogen (energy storehouses for future energy demands), but it also reduces insulin needs.

- Exercise increases insulin sensitivity in skeletal muscle for about forty-eight hours after exercising.

- Periods of inactivity lasting four to six days decrease insulin sensitivity (put another way, cause some insulin resistance).

- The more a person exercises, the better "trained" the cells are to dispose of glucose more efficiently. After just one exercise session, glucose disposal increases about 22 percent, but after six weeks of regular exercise, glucose disposal increases about 42 percent.

- Exercise probably changes the type of fiber in muscles to a type that is more insulin-sensitive. In addition, worked and trained muscles have a better blood supply and also have lower levels of fatty acids (that can contribute to insulin resistance).

Apple Shapes

A certain type of body fat is even more likely to cause insulin resistance: central obesity. This means excess fat around the midsection. We refer to people who carry their excess weight around the middle as apple shapes, while those who carry excess weight below the waist are pear shapes. Apple shapes are far more likely to get Type 2 diabetes than pear shapes. In fact, apple shapes who are only slightly overweight are at heightened risk for getting Type 2 diabetes because their fat cells are concentrated around the waist region.

You have probably guessed that it's time to get moving—whether or not you have Type 2 diabetes or not. Later chapters discuss exercise routines, including aerobic types and also resistance training (commonly called weight lifting).

Make sure that you always get a doctor's clearance before starting any new exercise routine, especially if you have been inactive or less active than you ought to be.

Chapter Two

Are You at Risk for Diabetes?

According to the Third National Health and Nutrition Examination Survey (a compilation of data gathered from 1988 to 1994), in the United States there is typically one undiagnosed case of Type 2 diabetes for each diagnosed case. The problems that go along with undiagnosed diabetes are as serious as those that go with diagnosed disease and often are more serious because blood sugar levels may be ranging out of control. In other words, hiding your head in the sand just doesn't work.

When blood sugars are even slightly high for a prolonged period, damage occurs in the heart, eyes, kidneys, nerves, and other organs of the body—*silently.* That is why it is so important to diagnose Type 2 diabetes early and treat it aggressively. Better yet, if you are at risk, you will learn from this book how to prevent it altogether and avoid the potentially disastrous complications.

Screening Tests for Diabetes

In 1998 the American Diabetes Association set new guidelines for the screening and diagnosis of Type 2 diabetes. One of the real tragedies of undiagnosed diabetes is that testing is so easy. Health care providers use three methods to screen for diabetes:

1. Fasting plasma glucose (FPG) test: This blood test is taken after fasting for at least eight hours; that is, having nothing to eat or drink for eight hours beforehand except water. This test is easy to perform and takes as long as it takes to draw blood.

2. Two-hour postprandial blood sugar test: Blood is drawn two hours after you eat. At one time diabetes specialists didn't pay much attention to this test, but it is taking on increasing importance. *We now know that postprandial, or after eating, blood sugars can reveal Type 2 diabetes even before the fasting blood sugar becomes abnormal.*

3. Oral glucose tolerance test (OGTT): This test takes longer and involves several blood tests taken within a certain number of minutes of each other and after drinking a specific sugary drink designed especially for the test.

Your health care provider will determine which test is best for you, but you can request both the fasting blood sugar test and the two-hour postprandial blood sugar test if you feel that it is warranted.

When Should I Be Screened for Diabetes?

You're probably going to think I am a stuck record, but you will see certain critical facts repeated several times in this chapter and elsewhere. One of the most important things to know comes from the American Diabetes Association:

New guidelines recommend that everyone age 40 to 45 and over consider being tested for the disease every three years. People at high risk should consider being tested at a younger age.

If you answer yes to any of the following questions, you may need screening for Type 2 diabetes. If the results indicate that you should be screened, call your doctor today for an appointment. *Early detection can mean fewer complications.* (Also, if you are at a health fair that offers blood sugar screening, please take advantage of the free, quick test! While the test won't give you a final answer, it will help reveal risk.)

- Do you have a blood relative with any type of diabetes?
- For women: Did you have gestational diabetes (diabetes during pregnancy)?
- For women: Did you have a baby weighing 9 pounds or more at birth?

- Are you of one of the following races:
  - —African American (Black American women are 2.41 times more likely to develop Type 2 diabetes than white women, and black men are 1.47 times more likely than white men.)
  - —Hispanic American
  - —Asian American
  - —Native American
  - —Pacific Islander
- Have you been told that you have impaired glucose tolerance? (Your health care provider would have performed this test.)
- Have you had an impaired fasting glucose test? (Your health care provider would have performed this test.)
- Do you have hypertension or high blood pressure? (See the chart for what is normal.)
- Do you have a high total cholesterol level or a high LDL cholesterol level? (See the chart for what is normal.)
- Do you have high triglyceride levels? (See the chart for what is normal.)
- Are you obese—is your body mass index (BMI) 25 or greater? (See the BMI chart.)
- Are you 40 to 45 years of age or older? (The American Diabetes Association recommends that you have blood glucose levels checked at least every three years, and more often if you have other risk factors.)

If you answered yes to any of the above questions, take the following quiz to get a more detailed assessment of your risk. It was designed by the American Diabetes Association to assess the risk of Type 2 diabetes and is used with their permission.

To find if you are at risk, write in the points next to each statement that is TRUE for you. If the answer is not true for you, then enter "0" for that question.

1. My weight is equal to or above that listed in the chart on page 19.
   Yes = 5, No = 0 _____

2. I am under 65 years of age AND I get little or no exercise during a usual day. Yes = 5, No = 0 _____

3. I am between 45 and 64 years of age. Yes = 5, No = 0 _____

4. I am 65 years old or older. Yes = 9, No = 0 _____

5. I am a woman who has had a baby weighing more than 9 pounds at birth. Yes = 1, No = 0 _____

6. I have a sister or a brother with diabetes. Yes = 1, No = 0 _____

7. I have a parent with diabetes. Yes = 1, No = 0 _____

Total Score _____

Scoring 3–9 points: You are probably at low risk for having diabetes *now*. But don't just forget about it, especially if you are Hispanic/Latino, African American, American Indian, Asian American, or Pacific Islander. You may be at higher risk in the future.

Scoring 10 or more points: You are at high risk for having diabetes. Only your health care provider can determine if you have diabetes. See your health care provider soon and find out for sure.

Know Your Numbers

It is up to you to know the numbers that place you at risk of Type 2 diabetes; these numbers also describe heart disease risk. If any of your statistics are not on a par with these recommendations, then you should visit your physician for diabetes screening.

- Total cholesterol should be less than 200.
- LDL cholesterol should be less than 100.
- HDL cholesterol should be greater than 45 for men and greater than 55 for women.
- Triglycerides should be less than 150.
- Fasting blood glucose should be 65 to 110.
- Hemoglobin A1C should be 4.0 to 6.0 percent.
- Blood pressure should be less than 120/80.

AT-RISK WEIGHT CHART

Height (without shoes)	Weight (pounds without clothing)
4' 10"	129
4' 11"	133
5' 0"	138
5' 1"	143
5' 2"	147
5' 3"	152
5' 4"	157
5' 5"	162
5' 6"	167
5' 7"	172
5' 8"	177
5' 9"	182
5' 10"	188
5' 11"	193
6' 0"	199
6' 1"	204
6' 2"	210
6' 3"	216
6' 4"	221

If you weigh the same or more than the amount listed for your height, you may be at risk for diabetes. This chart is based on a measure called the Body Mass Index (BMI). The chart shows unhealthy weights for men and women age 35 or older at the listed heights. At-risk weights are lower for individuals under age 35.

Source: Diabetes Forecast, March 1999.

Are There Any Symptoms of Type 2 Diabetes?

The trouble is that there often aren't any symptoms, especially in the early stages. But as time goes on and blood sugars climb higher, here are some of the symptoms that signify the presence of this disease:

- Increased or more frequent need to urinate (called *polyuria*)
- Increased thirst (*polydipsia*)
- Unexplained or unintended weight loss
- Blurred vision

Screening Kids for Diabetes

As noted earlier, kids are now getting Type 2 diabetes, which is one reason that the old term "adult-onset diabetes" is no longer accurate. Let's take a look at the facts, which will help you understand why kids should be screened earlier:

- Recent research shows a surge in children diagnosed with Type 2 diabetes.
- In 1990 fewer than 4 percent of diabetes cases in children were Type 2. This number has risen to approximately 20 percent, varying from 8 percent to 45 percent depending on the age of the group studied.
- Approximately 85 percent of children diagnosed with Type 2 diabetes are obese.
- Diabetes is the seventh leading cause of death in the United States.
- Approximately 15.7 million people, or 5.9 percent of the population, have diabetes.

According to the American Diabetes Association, at-risk children should be screened beginning at age 10 and every two years thereafter. Who is at risk?

- Children and teens who are sedentary
- Children and teens who overeat or are overweight
- Children and teens who have a family history of diabetes, especially if they are overweight and/or sedentary
- Children and teens from minority populations, including Mexican Americans, African Americans, and Native Americans, especially if they are overweight and/or sedentary

How to help your kids and grandkids prevent Type 2 diabetes:

1. Assist them in developing a healthier and leaner way of eating so they can lose excess weight or grow into their weight, which means growing taller without gaining weight. Your good example is most important.

2. Be more active with them. Remember, if they have been heavy and inactive, they should start physical activity slowly so they do not get injured. Just as adults need a doctor's approval before becoming more active, so should kids who are very heavy—in fact, so should all kids.

3. Try to get them to cut back on TV, computer, and video game time—and trade it for more active time. Make a deal that they can have one hour of "electronic" time for one hour of "active" time.

4. Get everyone, including the kids, into the habit of "drinking no empty calories." Share these facts with them:
   a. Drinking a 12-ounce soft drink ("pop") is like eating nine teaspoons of sugar.
   b. Drinking 20 ounces of pop is like eating fifteen teaspoons of sugar.
   c. Downing an oversized pop (32 ounces) is like eating twenty-five teaspoons of sugar.
   d. Children (and adults, too) need nonfat milk, about one quart per day. Drinking one quart of nonfat milk instead of 2% milk saves 142 calories and 17 grams of fat.

5. Work on the junk food situation. Make a habit of bringing home snack foods that everyone can eat for life. This includes fruits, vegetables, and frozen fruit bars. Leave the chips, snack cakes, and candy bars in the store.

Chapter Three

How Diabetes Affects Your Heart and Blood Vessels

You can't talk about Type 2 diabetes without talking about the dangers to your heart and blood vessels. That's because heart disease is the leading cause of death for those with Type 2 diabetes, and the damage to other blood vessels can be almost as critical.

Let's take a look at some of the facts:

- People with diabetes are two to four times more likely to have heart disease.

- Diabetes increases death rates from heart disease two- to fourfold.

- People with diabetes are two to four times more likely to suffer a stroke.

As you may have guessed by now, eating to control diabetes must also accommodate ways to control—and, it is hoped, diminish or even eradicate—heart disease. Fortunately, you will learn as you read on that this translates into wonderfully interesting and delicious food on your plate. One more great piece of news: This way of eating also helps prevent cancer and some chronic illnesses—definitely a win-win situation.

Heart mechanics.   Let's take a quick look at the heart's job in your body. Actually, the heart is one part of a larger system, the circulatory system. The other main part is the blood vessels, of which there are two main types: arteries and veins.

First, let's talk about the heart part of this system. The heart is a big muscle with a huge job: It pumps oxygen-rich blood to every nook and cranny of the body. Without oxygen the body's cells cannot survive.

Oxygen-rich blood leaves the heart through arteries and eventually travels into smaller vessels called capillaries to get to every cell. Once the cells extract the oxygen (and other nutrients), the oxygen-depleted blood travels back to the heart via the veins. The blood then goes to the lungs where it picks up oxygen, then makes a quick turn back to the heart, where it starts its journey again.

The danger of damaged vessels. Damage to the blood vessels results in less oxygen and fewer nutrients reaching the cells. If the blood supply is chronically diminished, cells die and then eventually tissues die, too. Poor blood supply can cause organ damage. For example, when the blood vessels that supply the heart become damaged, a heart attack can occur. When the vessels that supply blood to the brain become damaged, a stroke can occur. In other cases, diminished blood supply to the feet can cause the loss of a toe or even the foot, and possibly the entire leg. (Narrowed blood vessels that don't allow enough blood to get to your legs and feet is called peripheral vascular disease.) As you know, people with diabetes have far more amputations than the average person.

Signs and Symptoms of Peripheral Vascular Disease

While most people know the signs and symptoms of heart disease, few know those associated with vessels clogged in the legs and feet. If you are diabetic, see your physician at once if you have any of these symptoms:

- Pain in the buttocks
- Pain in the back of the legs or thighs when you stand, walk, or exercise

What damages vessels. In addition to family history, which you cannot change, there are many things that you can control that can damage blood vessels, such as:

- Consistently high blood sugars
- High cholesterol and other abnormal blood fats
- High blood pressure
- Smoking cigarettes
- Eating foods with too much saturated fat and too much cholesterol
- Being overweight
- Not getting enough exercise and activity

Diabetes and Blood Fats

It is critically important to know how diabetes interacts with and worsens high blood pressure and blood fats. (Because heart disease is about more than just cholesterol, I frequently use the phrase "blood fats" instead of blood cholesterol.) Learning about these factors will help you understand how Type 2 diabetes impacts your risk of heart disease.

Before going into the details of how having Type 2 diabetes affects your blood fats, let's take a look at some blood fat basics. When people discuss issues of the heart, they often discuss only the cholesterol level. However, it's important to discuss all the fats in the bloodstream because they are all factors of good health. We'll start by looking at cholesterol (and related compounds) and triglycerides.

Cholesterol in the blood. It is important to distinguish between cholesterol in the blood and cholesterol in food. Indeed, one of the reasons the whole topic of cholesterol is confusing is that health care professionals don't do a good job of distinguishing between them. You may be one of many who have walked out of a health professional's office with the order: "Watch your cholesterol." To be frank, that directive is absolutely meaningless.

25

Does that order mean you should watch the cholesterol you ingest from food, or does it mean do something about bringing your cholesterol level down? Who knows! But we do know that decreasing the amount of cholesterol you ingest is not the only thing you must do to reduce your risk of heart disease. In fact, reducing dietary cholesterol intake isn't even the most important action you can take. You will find a full discussion of dietary ways to bring down blood fat levels, including blood cholesterol levels, to healthier readings at the end of this chapter.

The word *cholesterol* tends to conjure up only negative thoughts, but we cannot live without some cholesterol in the body. It is such an important substance in the body that very little comes directly from ingested food. The liver makes most of it.

Cholesterol is an essential ingredient in many natural and normal body substances, including skin oils, hormones, digestive juices, and vitamin D. It is so necessary to good health that the body makes cholesterol in the liver. While we often refer to cholesterol as a fatty substance, it is really more of a waxy substance.

Cholesterol is carried around from one part of the body to another via the bloodstream. Just as oil and wax will not dissolve in water, waxy cholesterol by itself cannot dissolve in blood. To overcome this transportation problem, the liver becomes the packaging agent for cholesterol. Through a very complex process, the liver stuffs cholesterol into microscopic balls that are coated with protein shells. Protein dissolves in watery blood, which solves the problem of moving waxy cholesterol around in it. Now the cholesterol can travel through the blood from one part of the body to another. These cholesterol-containing, protein-coated little balls have a name: lipoproteins.

The significance of lipoproteins. The way cholesterol is packaged plays a more critical role than just moving cholesterol particles through the blood: It determines how cholesterol affects the health of the blood vessels through which it travels and, ultimately, the heart. Here's why:

There are four main types of protein shells. Shells with the least amount of protein are called very low density lipoproteins, or VLDLs. They have room for a lot of cholesterol. You probably haven't heard much about VLDLs because they don't stay in the bloodstream very long (although they take on a greater significance in people who have Type 2 diabetes). Nevertheless, they are potentially sinister because they contain large amounts of cholesterol and triglycerides, and have great potential to adhere to the arteries in the form of fatty plaque.

The lipoproteins that get the most attention are the low-density lipoproteins (LDLs). LDLs are very predictive of heart disease risk and are measured when you have a cholesterol test done. You have probably heard LDLs called "bad" cholesterol. Like VLDLs, LDLs with their high content of triglycerides and cholesterol are more likely to adhere to arterial walls as fatty plaque, thereby lodging in and blocking arteries—and instigating or contributing to atherosclerosis, or hardening of the arteries.

The story of artery-clogging LDLs gets worse. LDL cholesterol is susceptible to oxidative damage by oxygen-free radicals. Oxygen-free radicals are a fact of life. They are formed during the process of using oxygen in the body; they also come from cigarette smoke and exposure to too much sunlight.

While the body has a naturally occurring antioxidant defense system, it may not be enough to protect the arteries. You see, when LDL particles plop themselves on your artery walls, they are like magnets for oxygen-free radicals. When the free radicals attack the LDL particles on your artery walls, they make a bad situation even worse. The plaque surface becomes rough, and this roughened surface tries to repair itself, sending in scab-making material. (This is analogous to when a child falls and scrapes his knees. The roughened surface repairs itself when the body sends in scab-making material.) As you can imagine, this only further narrows the arteries. In addition, tiny pieces of the scab can break off, travel downstream, and lodge in even more narrowed areas. This may be what causes a heart attack or a stroke if it travels into the vessels that supply blood to the brain.

Now let's talk about the "good" high-density lipoproteins, or HDLs. HDLs have protein shells that are heavier and thicker, and therefore there is less room on the inside for cholesterol. Think of HDLs as the good guys who come to move cholesterol and other fats out of the bloodstream, to be shuttled out of the body by the liver. That is why HDL cholesterol is called the "good" cholesterol.

How do all of these things fit together? We run into heart health problems when there is too much total cholesterol in the bloodstream and when the ratio of LDL to HDL cholesterol is high. Knowing that LDLs are bad and HDLs good, it is easy to understand that heart troubles arise when too much cholesterol gets packaged as LDL particles. This also helps us appreciate why we need to know more than just our total cholesterol level.

What About Triglycerides?

There is one more factor we need to consider: triglycerides, the basic fat unit in the body. If we eat excess calories from any source—whether it is carbohydrates, protein, or fat—our bodies make triglycerides. When we really overeat, the excess triglycerides circulate in the bloodstream until they are stored as fat. Drinking alcohol can also cause the liver to produce excessive amounts of triglycerides.

Triglyceride levels are elevated when enzymes responsible for breaking down fats in the bloodstream are less active. This decreased enzyme activity results in higher VLDL and lower HDL levels, both of which are strongly associated with cardiovascular disease and heart attacks. This decreased enzyme activity might also cause harmful VLDL and smaller, dense LDL particles to circulate longer in the bloodstream.

The American Heart Association (AHA) says that triglyceride blood levels may be more predictive of heart attack risk than previously thought. Results of a study led by J. Michael Gaziano, M.D., director of cardiovascular epidemiology at Brigham and Women's Hospital in Boston, helps solidify the importance of triglycerides in predicting heart attack risk.

The findings of Gaziano's recent study suggest that a high ratio of triglycerides to HDL could prove to be a valuable marker for abnormal triglyceride metabolism as well as heart attack risk. "The ratio of triglycerides to HDL was the strongest predictor of a heart attack," said Gaziano. Compared with the lowest triglyceride/HDL ratios, those with the highest had a sixteenfold greater risk of a heart attack.

Why does diabetes greatly increase your risk of having atherosclerosis, or artery-clogging heart disease? The series of events that lead to atherosclerosis in people with Type 2 diabetes is very complex. People with Type 2 diabetes are more likely to have higher levels of triglycerides and lower levels of HDL cholesterol than those who don't have Type 2 diabetes.

The more their glucose levels range out of control, the higher their triglyceride levels climb. This situation is worse in people who are heavy.

There is at least one other reason that triglycerides climb in people with uncontrolled Type 2 diabetes. As you have learned by now, fat cells in people with Type 2 diabetes are prone to release free fatty acids. Among the negative consequences of free fatty acids, the body responds by producing an oversupply of very low density lipoproteins, or VLDLs. In turn, this causes the liver to make too many triglycerides. At the same time, the body's normal disposal mechanism for VLDLs is impaired, thereby causing these levels to rise ever more quickly.

One more critical fact to know: In diabetics who have central adiposity, or fat that accumulates in the midsection, these problems with triglycerides and VLDLs are accentuated.

Even with treatment for abnormal cholesterol levels, triglyceride levels can remain high and HDL cholesterol levels low. Other abnormalities may develop: LDL particles may become very small and very dense—definitely not a good thing because it makes them more sinister. Also, HDL composition may become abnormal, making it less of the good guy it is supposed to be.

When Type 2 diabetes is not under control, the body is less able to dispose of those bad LDL particles. Normally, the liver has a very sophisticated manner of filtering out excess LDL particles—it makes lipoprotein lipase. To put it simply, think of the liver as having grappling hooks that snare LDL particles, corral them, and send them out through the digestive tract. However, this filtering system is greatly impaired in Type 2 diabetes.

I stress again the cause of these blood fat abnormalities: Insulin resistance and central adiposity, and the two, of course, are related. Even if your pancreas manages to pump out enough insulin to keep blood sugars normal, these blood fat abnormalities can occur. That is why those who have insulin resistance before they are actually diagnosed with Type 2 diabetes—which is the case with most people—already have a greater risk of heart disease.

Now for some good news: Losing weight improves insulin resistance, and less insulin resistance means fewer blood fat abnormalities.

The message you should take away from all this is one of hope: You can do something about what causes your blood fat abnormalities. In fact, you can wipe them out (except those caused by your genetic makeup) by adopting the changes in lifestyle I will describe in great detail in this book.

Know Your Numbers

It is up to you to know the numbers that describe heart disease risk. The following are the desirable laboratory values for reducing heart disease risk. All the values shown here are for people with Type 2 diabetes. (The requirements are more stringent than for people who don't have diabetes.)

- Total cholesterol should be less than 200 mg/dl.
- LDL cholesterol should be less than 100 mg/dl.
- HDL cholesterol should be greater than 45 mg/dl for men and greater than 55 mg/dl for women.
- Triglycerides should be less than 150 mg/dl.
- Fasting blood glucose should be 65 to 110 mg/dl.
- Hemoglobin A1C should be 4.0 to 6.0 percent.
- Blood pressure should be less than 120/80 mmHg.

How Do I Keep Blood Cholesterol and Other Blood Fats at Healthy Normal Levels?

You will soon see that the diet I prescribe to control and eliminate high blood sugars is the same as the one to reduce your risk of heart disease. This is wonderful because you can keep one focus and be assured that your health will improve. (Note also that this diet will help prevent cancer and other chronic diseases, so you will need no other dietary advice.)

Here are your goals to keep blood fats at the healthiest reading possible:

Goal #1: Lose excess weight.

Goal #2: Control blood sugars.

Goal #3: Eat less fat and especially less saturated fat. (You will learn how in Chapter Six.)

Goal #4: Eat foods high in fiber, especially soluble fiber. (Chapter Four has many suggestions on getting fiber into your daily eating plan.)

Goal #5: Eat plenty of fruits, vegetables, legumes, and whole grains, which are high in vitamins, minerals, fiber, and phytochemicals. (You will find more about these substances and the role they play in heart disease and diabetes in Chapter Four as well as how to include them in every meal.)

Goal #6: Diversify your protein sources. Rather than rotating your eating of chicken, beef, and pork, make a point of including two or three fish meals per week and at least one vegetarian source of protein at dinner. In addition, try to make the protein at most lunch meals vegetarian types or include more fish. (Chapter Six contains detailed information about proteins and how you can incorporate the various sources into a healthy diet. Protein intake is closely tied to fat intake, which is why optimal fat intake is discussed in Chapter Five, before protein intake.)

Goal #7: Get moving. The human body is meant to be active, especially for the heart's sake. The heart is a muscular pump. Like any other muscle, the heart needs adequate exercise. If just getting up and walking around exercises the heart muscle, imagine what a brisk walk or using an exercise bicycle can do for it! Exercise confers many other significant benefits to the heart, including fighting the body's tendency to form tiny clots in the bloodstream—which can eventually coalesce into a larger clot that can cause a heart attack. Exercise also raises the good cholesterol, the high-density lipoprotein (HDL) cholesterol, which protects the heart. Engaging in regular exercise helps you manage stress and anger, which can otherwise contribute to increasing coronary artery disease (CAD) risk. (Chapter Seven gives more detailed information on exercise, why it is so important to you, and how to get moving safely.)

Understanding Blood Pressure

Your blood pressure reading has two numbers: the systolic (top) number and the diastolic (bottom) number. The systolic pressure is the pressure of blood against blood vessel walls when the heart contracts to squeeze blood out. The diastolic pressure is the pressure on the vessel walls between beats when the heart is at rest.

Hypertension

- Optimal blood pressure is below 120 systolic and 80 diastolic.

- High normal blood pressure is defined as between 130–139/85–89. A critically important fact here is that high normal blood pressure is of tremendous concern. An alarming one-third of all heart attacks and strokes occur in people with high normal blood pressure.

- A person has hypertension when pressures are over 140/90.

Why is hypertension more common and more dangerous in diabetics?   About 50 percent of people with diabetes also have hypertension. A person with diabetes and hypertension has more than seven times the expected rate of dying prematurely than others of his or her age. For someone with diabetes, hypertension, and some type of diabetic kidney disease (such as diabetic nephropathy), the risk of dying prematurely skyrockets to thirty-seven times the expected rate for that age. Not a pretty picture.

Why do people with Type 2 diabetes have more hypertension? There are several complex reasons that relate to the whole system of checks and balances that controls blood pressure in the body. Many of these are hormonally controlled (but not the hormones we generally think of that affect sex drive and hot flashes) and extremely complex. What you should know is that insulin resistance, which in turn causes the body to retain more fluid, throws off this system. As you probably know, fluid retention often drives up blood pressure.

Another reason that Type 2 diabetes drives up blood pressure involves the microvascular complications—the damage to blood vessels—that they develop. Damaged blood vessels are less elastic and therefore are more inclined to have higher pressure.

And that's not all. Having Type 2 diabetes places you at greater risk of having atherosclerosis, or clogged vessels, as you have already read. When vessels are clogged, the size of the lumen (the opening inside the blood vessel) through which blood flows decreases. This causes increased pressure inside the vessels.

Here is an analogy to make the above concept clearer: Have you ever put your finger over the end of a garden hose when the water was flowing at full blast? It causes the water to come out at greatly increased pressure. Not only that but the pressure inside the hose is also substantially increased. This is what happens inside your vessels when the size of the opening decreases.

Carrying extra weight, independent of having Type 2 diabetes, also increases blood pressure. We know that a go-cart engine does not have enough energy to power a car. Unfortunately, the one-third of Americans who are seriously overweight demand a similar feat of their bodies every day. The heart just is not meant to pump hard enough to get blood to all the excess tissue day after day. The strain can result in high blood pressure.

As mentioned earlier, people with Type 2 diabetes are more likely to carry fat around their midsection even if they are not terribly overweight, and this fat reacts differently from fat in other parts of the body. For example, these central fat cells release more free fatty acids. Among other negative effects, these increased numbers of free fatty acids cause what is called vascular reactivity, which means they cause the walls of the blood vessels to contract much more than is normal and good. The end result is higher blood pressure.

What are the symptoms of hypertension? That's the problem! There generally aren't any symptoms. That is why hypertension is called the silent killer.

How do you control hypertension? The good news is that controlling diabetes, losing weight, and eating the health- and life-giving diet given in this book can bring hypertension under control and bring your risks down to normal. As you'll quickly notice, the goals for lowering blood pressure are just about identical to those for lowering cholesterol levels.

Goal #1: Lose excess weight. Yes, you've heard this theme before, but shedding the pounds will decrease insulin resistance. In turn, you'll suffer fewer microvascular complications and fewer abnormalities in that complex hormone system that controls blood pressure. In addition, the simple fact of losing weight decreases the stress of pumping blood throughout the body and also decreases blood pressure independently of the wonderfully positive changes that happen when blood sugars and insulin resistance improve.

Goal #2: Control blood sugars. Shedding pounds will also help you control blood sugars, which will decrease insulin resistance and cut down on the chemical changes that raise blood pressure.

Goal #3: Reduce sodium, but increase other salts. We know from the DASH study (Dietary Approaches to Stop Hypertension) that getting enough of certain critical minerals or salts is as important as decreasing the amount of the mineral you've heard most about: sodium (the blood-pressure-raising ingredient in table salt). DASH researchers found that those who consumed large quantities of fruits, vegetables, whole grains, legumes, and lean dairy, and who also decreased dietary fat substantially, had much lower blood pressure than people who ate quite differently in the study. One of the theories is that magnesium, potassium, and calcium—minerals or salts found in significant amounts in such an eating style—play important roles in lowering blood pressure.

Goal #4: Decrease blood cholesterol levels. You may think I'm beginning to sound repetitive, but as you learned above, decreasing blood cholesterol levels can help you avoid clogged and stiff arteries, and this decreases your chances of having high blood pressure.

Goal #5: Exercise regularly. Exercise has multiple benefits: It can help you achieve a leaner body, which can decrease blood sugar abnormalities, blood cholesterol levels, and also hypertension. (Chapter Seven offers details on the benefits of exercise.)

What About Alcohol and the Heart When You Have Diabetes?

You have probably heard that red wine is good for the heart. The truth is, the advice about alcohol and heart disease is quite complicated.

Perhaps the most important message about alcohol is that although a little may be good for the heart, too much increases cardiovascular problems, including heart rhythm abnormalities and heart failure. Too much is probably less than you think: Experts believe that anything more than one drink is probably too much. Population-based data clearly reveal that the benefit of alcohol is more evident among light to moderate drinkers.

The most popular theory concerning alcohol's ability to reduce heart disease focuses on HDL cholesterol. Alcohol seems to raise this good cholesterol, thereby helping to reduce cholesterol buildup on arterial walls. Another possibility is that alcohol decreases platelet aggregation or renders platelets less sticky and therefore less likely to clump together. Alcohol also seems to encourage the body to produce greater amounts of a clot-dissolving chemical called tissue plasminogen activator that helps break up the little clots that continuously form in the bloodstream.

Must It Be Red Wine?

The answer is probably no, but red wine may offer additional benefits over and above its alcohol intake. The red grapes from which red wine is made are high in flavonoids, one type of phytochemical or health-promoting plant substance. Flavonoids act as powerful antioxidants, which, among other actions, protect against heart disease. Fortunately, you do not have to imbibe an alcoholic beverage such as red wine to harvest flavonoids: A wide variety of fruits and vegetables offers rich amounts. Apples, onions, and green beans are among the flavonoid-rich choices; green and black teas are also very high in this phytochemical.

If you have diabetes, however, there is even more to discuss about alcohol intake. Alcohol can raise triglyceride levels, especially in people who have Type 2 diabetes. Another problem can occur in people who have diabetes and who take insulin or medications to control their blood sugars. Contrary to popular belief, alcohol actually decreases blood sugar levels. This is because alcohol inhibits the liver from making glucose. For the many hours that the alcohol remains in the body, no glucose enters the bloodstream from the liver. You get glucose only from the food you eat during the time you are drinking.

You should also know that the glucose-lowering effect of alcohol could last for as long as eight to twelve hours (remember, this is only a problem for people who take blood-sugar-lowering medications and/or insulin). Worse, the problems of abnormally low levels of glucose (hypoglycemia) occur at relatively low levels of intoxication. Unless the people you are with know you well, they are likely to misinterpret your signs of hypoglycemia as signs of intoxication and not realize that you should get some form of easily digestible carbohydrate into you right away, such as a glass of orange juice.

Needless to say, drinking alcohol when you have diabetes and take diabetic control medications can be very dangerous.

Here is good advice about alcohol:

- If you do not drink now, do not start in order to decrease your risk of heart disease. If you want to do something to reduce heart disease risk, choose something more powerful—such as a thirty-minute daily walk or reducing your saturated fat intake.

- If you drink now, stop at one drink. A drink is defined as 12 ounces of beer, 5 ounces of wine, or 1.5 ounces of hard liquor. (Women should note, however, that even this light-to-moderate level of alcohol consumption might increase breast cancer risk.) The calories alone in alcohol are enough to keep your weight up—as well as your insulin resistance.

- If you take medications or insulin to control blood glucose levels, never drink on an empty stomach. Make sure you eat before you go to a party where there is alcohol, and try to nibble throughout the evening.

- If you take medications or insulin, nurse one drink all evening. Sip it slowly to last the entire evening. Or after one drink, switch to club soda or diet soda. You'll feel better now—and in the future.

Why Smoking Is Slow Suicide

You can't discuss heart disease without discussing smoking. Inhaling tobacco smoke causes immediate negative effects on the heart and blood vessels in addition to long-term effects. The sinister impact is also cumulative. Some of these ill effects and reasons to stop smoking include the following:

An increase in heart rate: Within one minute of starting to smoke, the heart rate begins to rise; it may increase by as much as 30 percent during the first ten minutes of smoking.

- An acute increase in blood pressure: Blood vessels constrict, forcing the heart to work harder to deliver oxygen to the rest of the body and to the heart muscle itself. Smoking causes blood pressure variability, which is even more likely to lead to heart damage than regular high blood pressure, and it reduces the effectiveness of blood pressure medication.

- Compromised oxygen supply: One ingredient of tobacco smoke, carbon monoxide, exerts a negative effect on the heart by compromising the blood's ability to carry oxygen. For people with diabetes this is a great concern, especially if they have already suffered microvascular complications that impaired blood flow and oxygen delivery.

- In women, smoking is associated with an earlier menopause. The onset of menopause raises heart disease risk because at menopause women all but stop producing estrogen—and estrogen protects against heart disease. Even female smokers who have not yet reached menopause have lower than normal estrogen levels, another means by which smoking increases heart disease risk. Remember, if you have diabetes, you already have a significantly heightened risk of heart disease, so don't give yourself this double whammy.

Once you stop smoking, you'll also enjoy an improved sense of taste and smell, and you will look better physically (smoking causes face wrinkles, stained teeth, and dull skin).

How to stop smoking: The highly addictive nature of smoking makes quitting a difficult proposition. Behavioral experts say you can increase your chances of long-term success by starting with a plan. Before you quit, think through the following points and plan accordingly:

- Pick a date to stop smoking and then get ready for it.
- Record when and why you smoke. You will come to know what triggers your urges to smoke.
- Record what you do when you smoke. As you reduce the number of cigarettes you have each day, have them at different times and different

places than you used to when you smoked more. This helps break the connection between smoking and certain activities.

- List your reasons for quitting. Read over the list before and after you quit.
- Find activities to replace smoking. Be ready to do something else when you want to smoke.
- Ask your health care provider about using nicotine gum, patches, and inhalers. Some people find these aids very helpful.

Be aware of how you feel when you quit smoking. At first you will crave cigarettes, be irritable, feel very hungry, cough often, get headaches, or have difficulty concentrating. These symptoms of withdrawal occur because your body is used to nicotine, the active addicting agent in cigarettes.

When withdrawal symptoms occur during the first two weeks after quitting, stay in control. Think about your reasons for quitting. Remind yourself that these are signs your body is healing and getting used to being without cigarettes.

The withdrawal symptoms are only temporary. They are strongest when you first quit but will go away within ten to fourteen days. Remember that these symptoms are easier to treat than the major diseases that smoking can cause.

You may still have the desire to smoke because of strong associations, such as with certain people, with specific situations, or with a variety of emotions. The best way to overcome these associations is to experience them without smoking.

If you smoke again (called a relapse), do not lose hope. Seventy-five percent of smokers who quit relapse. Most smokers quit three times before they are successful. If you relapse, do not give up! Plan ahead and think about what you will do the next time you get the urge to smoke.

Chapter Four

What to Believe About Carbohydrates and Fiber

You are not alone if you're afraid of carbohydrates. You are also not alone if you are totally confused about carbohydrates. Indeed, there is no more confusing food topic than carbohydrates—not just for diabetics but for everyone.

One day we hear "Eat carbs and no fat." The next day we hear "Avoid all carbs and eat a high-protein diet." Yet another day we hear that we should eat only low-glycemic carbs.

Even if you didn't have diabetes, you would need some help in understanding this confusing concept of carbohydrates. To help you sort this out, I suggest you keep two things in mind as you read this chapter:

1. Carbohydrates are a calorie-containing nutrient.
2. There are carbohydrate-containing foods.

The two are not the same. Once you read this chapter you will understand why you need to eat about half of your calories as carbohydrates—but specific ones. (Don't worry. I'm going to help you understand which ones and why.) When you consume 50 to 60 percent of your daily calories as carbohydrate calories (from specific foods), you can better control Type 2 diabetes and reduce the risk of associated heart disease. The pattern in which you eat these carbohydrates is also very important to both controlling blood sugars and reducing heart disease risk.

The Role of Carbohydrates in Optimal Eating

In this section you will find a clear picture of carbohydrates and how they fit into the total scheme of a healthy eating plan. You will learn:

- how carbohydrates are made;
- the role carbohydrates play in the diet;
- why planning carbohydrate-rich foods is critical to controlling diabetes;
- why you need a healthy mix of carbohydrate foods.

How Mother Nature Makes Carbohydrates

The process starts with green plants. The plant's leaves "breathe in" carbon dioxide. (Interestingly enough, humans breathe in oxygen and exhale carbon dioxide as the waste product, and plants do just the opposite.) At the other end, in the roots, the plant absorbs water. With the energy that the plant absorbs from the sun, it breaks apart the water molecules into its constituent ingredients: hydrogen atoms and oxygen atoms. The hydrogen atoms combine with the carbon dioxide to make a basic sugar unit in what will soon become the edible portion of the plant, often called the fruit or the seed. We call this basic sugar unit a monosaccharide (*mono* means one).

Nature makes three basic types of monosaccharides, or one-unit sugars:

1. Galactose, one of the sugars found in milk
2. Glucose, one of the sugars found in fruits, vegetables, and honey
3. Fructose, one of the sugars found in fruits, artichokes, and honey

Mother Nature joins two sugar units together to form a disaccharide (*di* means two). The following are some of the disaccharides found in food:

- Maltose: two units of glucose joined together; these are particularly abundant in germinated grains.
- Sucrose: formed from one unit of fructose and one of glucose; sugar beets and the sap of sugar maple trees are rich in sucrose.

- Lactose: formed from a unit of glucose plus one of galactose; lactose is unique to milk.

Both mono- and disaccharides dissolve in the watery juices of plants, which facilitates their transport from one part of the plant to another. Some of these mono- and disaccharides are tucked away in the juice of plants for later uses, but the majority join together to form larger units called polysaccharides (*poly* means many).

Polysaccharides are sugars formed from hundreds or thousands of monosaccharides and disaccharides joined together. Foods high in polysaccharides are called starches or complex carbohydrates. Examples of starchy foods include whole grain foods, potatoes, legumes (such as black beans), and rice.

Carbohydrates Are Just One Type of Calorie

Now let's look at how carbohydrates fit into the total scheme of nutrition that our bodies need.

Mother Nature made food with three basic types of life-giving and health-promoting substances:

1. Macronutrients, of which there are two main types: water and energy-containing substances
2. Micronutrients, of which there are two main types: vitamins and minerals
3. Phytochemicals, or plant chemicals, which are thought to promote good health by helping to reduce the risk of heart disease, cancer, and other chronic diseases. There are thousands of different types of phytochemicals in plant foods (see the sidebar for a brief explanation).

As you probably know by now, the majority of foods are a combination of all these things. And as you will read repeatedly in this book, foods that pack in the greatest number of substances—vitamins, minerals, and phytochemicals—are the most valuable to us and our health.

Let's now concentrate on energy-containing substances—known as *calories*. Foods can contain three basic types of calories: carbohydrates, proteins, and fats (there is actually a fourth, alcohol, but we don't consider that

Phytochemicals

Phytochemicals have taken nutrition science to the next level. The word means plant chemicals (the Greek prefix *phyto* means plant). The most visible function of phytochemicals is to give plants their range of brilliant rainbow colors. They also serve as the natural defense mechanism of plants. For instance, an insect that bites into a garlic clove will quickly buzz away because of the putrid smell and taste. Similarly, phytochemicals work well to fight off viruses, molds, and bacteria that can harm plants.

But in the last decade of the last century nutrition scientists discovered that phytochemicals have value for human health. Many phytochemicals are powerful antioxidants that help to fight cancer and heart disease. Phytochemicals also offer health benefits beyond their antioxidant power.

The fascinating thing about phytochemicals is that they generally travel in colors. That is why nutritionists advise everyone to eat at least three to five different colors of fruits and vegetables per day. You are then assured of getting the wide array of phytochemicals we need to protect our health.

One example of a class of phytochemicals you may have heard of is flavonoids. Several studies have shown that people who eat foods rich in flavonoids, as part of an overall healthy eating plan, decrease their risk of heart attack and stroke.

a macronutrient needed for good health). Most foods are composed of some combination of these three types of calories (although certain foods, such as oils, contain all fat calories, and table sugar contains all carbohydrate calories). Here are some examples:

- Skim milk: 56 percent of its calories come from carbohydrates, 33 percent from protein, and 5 percent from fat.

- Oatmeal: 69 percent of its calories come from carbohydrates, 17 percent from protein, and 14 percent from fat.

- Walnuts: 7 percent of its calories come from carbohydrates, 15 percent from protein, and 78 percent from fat.

- Salmon: 0 calories come from carbohydrates, 58 percent from protein, and 42 percent from fat.

- Plain bagel: 79 percent of its calories come from carbohydrates, 16 percent from protein, and 5 percent from fat.

- Pretzels: 88 percent of their calories come from carbohydrates and 12 percent from protein.

- Lentils: 67 percent of its calories come from carbohydrates, 30 percent from protein, and 3 percent from fat.

The above examples should help you realize one very important thing: There is a wide world of carbohydrate-containing foods out there. Even more important, your body needs many of these foods for good health and to control your diabetes. Sadly, if you are trying to avoid carbohydrate-containing foods because of some recent fad advice, you will miss out on these wonderful foods.

In fact, cutting back on carbohydrate-containing foods backfires greatly on people with Type 2 diabetes. Research has shown that meals with a low carbohydrate content spur the body to pump out high levels of free fatty acids. And as I've said before, *free fatty acids are not good*. They cause insulin resistance and the long chain of bad events that follows.

Even Distribution of Carbohydrate Calories Is Critical to Controlling Diabetes

While the majority of your calories should come from carbohydrates, it is critical to plan which ones and the pattern in which you eat them. Let me simplify this critically important point with a couple of explanatory points:

While there are three types of calories—carbohydrates, proteins, and fats—only one contributes to raising your blood sugar: carbohydrates.

Carbohydrate calories (and therefore carbohydrate-containing foods) should be distributed evenly throughout the day to help control rises in blood sugar. To be more explicit, you should have some at breakfast, some as a morning snack, some at lunch, some as an afternoon snack, and some at dinner. Giving your body smaller carbohydrate portions at one time is key to preventing huge increases in blood sugar. By having carbohydrate portions throughout the day, many people can successfully control Type 2 diabetes without medication.

Foods that contain carbohydrate calories bring value to our health for many other reasons, which leads us to the next point.

Types of Carbohydrate-Containing Foods and Why You Need Them All

There is a vast world of carbohydrate-containing foods out there. There are five main categories of carbohydrate-containing foods that should be part of a healthy eating plan:

1. Fruits
2. Vegetables
3. Legumes, such as black beans, lentils, and kidney beans
4. Whole grains and whole grain foods, such as bread, oatmeal, rice, barley, and whole grain bread
5. Nonfat and low-fat dairy foods, such as skim milk, nonfat yogurt, and low-fat yogurt

Including all these types of carbohydrates in your daily eating plan is key to achieving good health. We will look at a couple of foods in each category and discover the life-giving and health-promoting substances that are unique to each category.

For the sake of comparison, I've tallied the nutritional content of about 80 to 100 calories of each food. This will help give you some concept of how nutritionally powerful certain foods are; this is called "nutrient density." The terms

Daily Value and *Percent Daily Value (% Daily Value* or *% DV)* are used on the nutrition labels of food products.

Daily Values are set by the government and reflect current nutrition recommendations for a 2,000-calorie diet. The % Daily Value can be used to compare food products and see how the amount of a nutrient in a serving of food fits into a 2,000-calorie diet.

A Look at Some Fruits

Fresh pear (medium size, about 6 ounces whole)
- 100 calories, 88 percent of which are carbohydrates
- 4 grams fiber
- The bonus of:
    11% DV vitamin C
    9% DV copper
    6% DV manganese
    6% DV potassium

Two fresh peaches (each medium size; the two together weigh 7 ounces total)
- 84 calories, 92 percent of which are carbohydrates
- 4 grams fiber
- The bonus of:
    11% DV vitamin A
    5% DV riboflavin
    10% DV niacin
    22% DV vitamin C
    7% DV vitamin E
    7% DV copper
    5% DV manganese
    11% DV potassium

Two fresh kiwifruits (total weight 5.5 ounces before peeling)
- 92 calories, 85 percent of which are carbohydrates
- 5 grams fiber

- The bonus of:
    - 5% DV vitamin A
    - 190% DV vitamin C
    - 9% DV vitamin E
    - 12% DV copper
    - 11% DV magnesium
    - 8% DV manganese
    - 6% DV phosphorus
    - 14% DV potassium

Fresh banana (medium size, about 4 ounces before peeling)
- 108 calories, 92 percent of which are carbohydrates
- 3 grams fiber
- The bonus of:
    - 7% DV riboflavin
    - 34% DV vitamin B_6
    - 18% DV vitamin C
    - 6% DV folate
    - 6% DV copper
    - 9% DV magnesium
    - 9% DV manganese
    - 13% DV potassium

A Look at Some Starchier Vegetables

Baked potato, served with the skin (about 3 ounces in weight after baking)
- 92 calories, 91 percent of which are carbohydrates
- 2 grams fiber
- The bonus of:
    - 2 grams protein
    - 6% DV thiamin
    - 7% DV niacin
    - 15% DV vitamin B_6

> 18% DV vitamin C
> 5% DV pantothenic acid
> 13% DV copper
> 6% DV iron
> 6% DV magnesium
> 10% DV manganese
> 5% DV phosphorus
> 10% DV potassium

Baked sweet potato (about 3 ounces of flesh after baking)
- 87 calories, 93 percent of which are carbohydrates
- 2.5 grams fiber
- The bonus of:
> 371% DV vitamin A
> 6% DV riboflavin
> 10% DV vitamin B_6
> 35% DV vitamin C
> 5% DV folate
> 6% DV pantothenic acid
> 9% DV copper
> 24% DV manganese
> 5% DV phosphorus
> 8% DV potassium

⅔ cup peas (cooked from frozen)
- 83 calories, 71 percent of which are carbohydrates
- 6 grams fiber
- The bonus of:
> 14% DV vitamin A
> 20% DV thiamin
> 6% DV riboflavin
> 8% DV niacin
> 6 % DV vitamin B_6
> 18% DV vitamin C

16% DV folate

7% DV copper

9% DV iron

8% DV magnesium

22% DV manganese

10% DV phosphorus

7% DV zinc

A Look at Some Less Starchy Vegetables

3 large carrots

- 93 calories, 87 percent of which are carbohydrates
- 6.5 grams fiber
- For the bonus of:

  2 grams protein

  270% DV vitamin A

  14% DV thiamin

  7% DV niacin

  16% DV vitamin B_6

  33% DV vitamin C

  5% DV vitamin E

  8% DV folate

  392% DV vitamin K

  6% DV calcium

  5% DV copper

  6% DV iron

  8% DV magnesium

  15% DV manganese

  14% DV molybdenum

  10% DV phosphorus

  20% DV potassium

3 sweet red bell peppers

- 96 calories, 83 percent of which are carbohydrates

- 7 grams fiber
- The bonus of:
    - 3 grams protein
    - 203% vitamin A
    - 16% DV thiamin
    - 6% DV riboflavin
    - 9% DV niacin
    - 44% DV vitamin B_6
    - 1131% DV vitamin C
    - 12% DV vitamin E
    - 20% DV folate
    - 12% DV copper
    - 9% DV iron
    - 9% DV magnesium
    - 21% DV manganese
    - 7% DV phosphorus
    - 18% DV potassium

4 cups raw broccoli florets

- 80 calories, 58 percent of which are carbohydrates
- 8.5 grams protein
- The bonus of:
    - 8.5 grams protein
    - 44% DV vitamin A
    - 12% DV thiamin
    - 20% DV riboflavin
    - 23% DV vitamin B_6
    - 441% DV vitamin C
    - 24% DV vitamin E
    - 50% DV folate
    - 15% DV pantothenic acid
    - 14% DV calcium
    - 14% DV iron
    - 18% DV magnesium

33% DV manganese

19% DV phosphorus

25% DV potassium

12% DV selenium

8% DV zinc

A Look at Some Grain Foods

⅓ cup cooked barley

- 90 calories, 83 percent of which are carbohydrates
- 4.5 grams fiber
- The bonus of:
    2.5 grams protein
    11% DV copper
    10% DV manganese
    8% DV phosphorus
    17% DV selenium

½ cup cooked oatmeal

- 96 calories, 69 percent of which are carbohydrates
- 2.6 grams fiber
- The bonus of:
    4 grams protein
    11% DV thiamin
    6% DV iron
    9% DV magnesium
    46% DV manganese
    12% DV phosphorus
    18% DV selenium
    5% DV zinc

⅔ cup cooked bulgur

- 100 calories, 84 percent of which are carbohydrates
- 5.5 grams fiber

- The bonus of:
    4 grams protein
    5% DV thiamin
    6% DV niacin
    5% DV vitamin B$_6$
    5% DV folate
    5% DV copper
    6% DV iron
    10% DV magnesium
    37% DV manganese
    5% DV phosphorus
    5% DV zinc

⅔ **cup cooked corn** (yes, corn is a grain!)
- 88 calories, 46 percent of which are carbohydrates
- 2 grams fiber
- The bonus of:
    3 grams protein
    5% DV riboflavin
    7% DV niacin
    15% DV vitamin C
    13% DV folate
    5% DV iron
    5% DV magnesium
    9% DV manganese
    7% DV phosphorus
    6% DV potassium

A Look at Legumes

½ **cup cooked black beans**
- 113 calories, 70 percent of which are carbohydrates
- 7.5 grams fiber

- The bonus of:
    7.6 grams protein
    14% DV thiamin
    32% DV folate
    9% DV copper
    10% DV iron
    15% DV magnesium
    19% DV manganese
    12% DV phosphorus
    9% DV potassium
    6% DV zinc

½ cup cooked lentils

- 114 calories, 67 percent of which are carbohydrates
- 8 grams fiber
- The bonus of:
    9 grams protein
    11% DV thiamin
    9% DV vitamin B_6
    45% DV folate
    6% DV pantothenic acid
    12% DV copper
    18% DV iron
    9% DV magnesium
    24% DV manganese
    18% DV phosphorus
    10% DV potassium
    8% DV zinc

A Look at Dairy Foods

(Cheeses are discussed in the protein chapter because they contain few carbohydrates.)

1 cup or 8 ounces skim milk
- 85 calories, 56 percent of which are carbohydrates
- 0 fiber
- The bonus of:
    - 8.5 grams protein
    - 15% DV vitamin A
    - 20% DV riboflavin
    - 15% DV vitamin B_{12}
    - 25% DV vitamin D
    - 30% DV calcium
    - 25% DV phosphorus
    - 12% DV potassium
    - 7% DV selenium
    - 7% DV zinc

1 cup or 8 ounces whole milk
- 149 calories, 30 percent of which are carbohydrates
- 0 fiber
- While the nutrient bonuses are similar to skim milk, you are also getting several negatives:
    - 49 percent of calories are fat calories
    - 5 grams of artery-clogging saturated fat
    - 33 grams cholesterol

1 cup or 8 ounces nonfat yogurt
- 100 calories, 66 percent of which are carbohydrates
- 0 fiber
- The bonus of:
    - 10 grams protein
    - 20% DV riboflavin
    - 15% DV vitamin B_{12}
    - 10% DV pantothenic acid
    - 30% DV calcium

23% DV phosphorus

11% DV potassium

10% DV zinc

1 cup or 8 ounces whole milk yogurt

- 150 calories, 30 percent of which are carbohydrates
- 0 fiber
- While the nutrient bonuses are similar to nonfat yogurt, you are also getting several negatives:

    47 percent of calories are fat calories

    5 grams of artery-clogging saturated fat

    31 grams cholesterol

½ cup nonfat cottage cheese

- 80 calories, 21 percent of which are carbohydrates
- 0 fiber
- The bonus of:

    15 grams fiber

    10% DV riboflavin

    10% DV vitamin B$_{12}$

    6% DV calcium (if you choose calcium fortified, this goes up considerably)

    15% DV phosphorus

½ cup 4% fat cottage cheese

- 120 calories, 14 percent of which are carbohydrates
- 0 fiber
- While the nutrient bonuses are similar to nonfat cottage cheese, you are also getting several negatives:

    38 percent of calories are fat calories

    3.5 grams of artery-clogging saturated fat

    25 grams cholesterol

What Have These Examples Taught Us?

The first thing you probably noticed is that every food, no matter how similar it seems to another, offers an entirely different array of nutrients. That is why nutrition experts advise everyone to eat a variety of different foods every day.

This point is very important. Eating a wide variety of foods has been called the "whole-diet approach." In the April 26, 2000, issue of the *Journal of the American Medical Association,* researchers from the Department of Family, Nutrition and Exercise Sciences at Queens College of the City University of New York reported the results of their study concerning the health effects of eating a larger number of foods. They found that what we eat really does affect our health and that focusing on the total diet, rather than on individual nutrients, is the key to better health.

For this study researchers spent about fifteen years tracking the health status and death rates of more than forty-two thousand women whose average age was 61. About halfway through the study the women completed a questionnaire asking which of sixty-two foods they had eaten in the past year. The researchers then selected twenty-three foods from the list that fit into the dietary guidelines, or the food pyramid, and measured the women's diet quality by counting how many of these twenty-three foods each woman ate at least once a week. From that information they calculated food scores that were adjusted to account for differences in age, race, education, smoking status, alcohol consumption, weight, total calories consumed, physical activity level, and other health factors. The researchers divided the women into four groups based on food scores. They found that the women with the highest scores (14 to 23) had about a 30 percent lower risk of dying from any cause than those with the lowest scores (0 to 8). Looking at specific causes of death, the researchers found that women with the highest scores were 40 percent less likely to die of cancer, 33 percent less likely to die of heart disease, and 42 percent less likely to die of stroke than women in the poorest quality diet group.

This study shows that ordinary people can achieve diets healthy enough to prolong their lives. This book is going to help you learn to make this wider variety of choices.

Now, back to our glimpse into foods. Different groups of carbohydrate-rich foods generally contribute a unique profile of nutrients, as follows:

- Fruits are rich in fiber, vitamin A, vitamin C, folate, potassium, and often vitamin E.
- Vegetables contribute fiber, protein, vitamin A, vitamin C, often vitamin E, potassium, and a wider variety of minerals than fruits.
- Whole grains and grain foods are rich in fiber (some in soluble fiber), protein, and some B vitamins, and are very rich in minerals.
- Legumes are an excellent source of protein, fiber (especially soluble fiber), folate, potassium, iron, and several minerals.
- Dairy foods are excellent sources of protein, vitamin D, calcium, phosphorus, potassium, riboflavin, and vitamin B_{12}. Notice, however, the huge difference in fat, saturated fat, and cholesterol content between the two types of dairy foods, those with fat and those without. If you compare a glass of skim milk with a glass of whole fat milk, and so on, you will see that you benefit significantly from including the nonfat dairy (and lower fat cheese).

That "Other" Category of Carbohydrate-Containing Foods

Foods in this category are the ones that cause most of the confusion about eating carbohydrate-containing foods. In fact, these are the foods that give all carbohydrate-containing foods a bad reputation. I call this category *simplified, stripped-of-nutrients, carbohydrate-containing foods.*

Here are some examples to help you understand why it isn't a good idea to include these foods in your diet with any regularity.

Soda pop or soft drinks and other sugary beverages
- Fruit Punch Sports Drink, 12 ounces
    - 85 calories, 100 percent of which are carbohydrates
    - 0 fiber
    - 0 protein

- For the bonus of:

   Nothing. There is no nutrient contribution of at least 5% DV except for sodium.

Snack items such as cookies and chips

- 3 vanilla wafer cookies

   78 calories, 67 percent of which are carbohydrates and 27 percent of which are fat; 7 percent of those fat calories are artery-clogging saturated fat

   0 fiber

   1.2 grams protein

- For the bonus of:

   Nothing. There is no nutrient contribution of at least 5% DV.

- 25 tiny cheese-flavored, fish-shaped crackers:

   64 calories, 53 percent of which are carbohydrates and 37 percent of which are fat; 10 percent of those are artery-clogging saturated fat

   0 fiber

   1.5 grams protein

- For the bonus of:

   88 grams cholesterol (which is not good)

   Trans fatty acids (not good either)

   6% DV thiamin (because fortified white flour was used to make them)

Here is the impression you should retain of these foods: Through extensive processing in the food manufacturing process, they no longer resemble what Mother Nature made. Now they are calorically dense and have very little of the wonderful life-giving substances tucked in by Mother Nature. If you use the food in the form in which it came to us from Mother Nature, you'll be one giant step closer to good health.

In years gone by, diabetes experts recommended that people with diabetes avoid sugar. According to the American Diabetes Association, it was assumed that sugar, which quickly changes into glucose, would raise blood glucose levels more. But research has shown that this is not true. Nevertheless, there are other reasons to slash the amount of sugary items in your eating plan. You have learned that sugary items:

- are calorically dense or contribute a large number of calories in a small amount of food (take a look at the fruit punch example);
- offer little appetite-holding power because they have no fiber or protein. As a result you end up searching for food again soon after ingesting them;
- contribute nothing to your nutritional profile except calories. This means you have fewer calories left for foods that your body craves for good health.

Fiber: Essential Threads of Good Health

You may have noticed one common thread of the first group of carbohydrate-rich foods discussed above: They all contribute significant amounts of fiber. Fiber can be very helpful to you as a person with Type 2 diabetes for three reasons. It may help slow the rise in blood glucose after a meal, it may help decrease the insulin response after eating, and it may help lower your LDL or bad cholesterol level.

What Is Fiber?

The number one thing to know about fiber is that it is found only in foods that come from plants. This includes four of those wonderful categories of carbohydrate-containing foods discussed above: fruits, vegetables, whole grains, and legumes; dairy foods don't have fiber because they are animal products.

The fiber in plants is somewhat like the fibers or threads that form clothing. Just as threads give cloth structure, fiber lends structure and strength to plants. Owing partly to this strength, fibers in fruits and vegetables are indigestible, which means our bodies cannot break them down. These fibers literally add bulk to intestinal waste products, which is why fiber-containing foods are often called bulky foods.

Just as there is more than one type of thread to make cloth, there are many types of fibers found in plants, and they are divided into two main types: insoluble and soluble. Insoluble fiber soaks up water much as a sponge would, making stools softer and easier to eliminate. Many vegetables, wheat bran, and other whole grains are good sources of insoluble fiber.

In contrast, soluble fiber dissolves in the watery contents of the gastrointestinal tract to form a gel. Soluble fiber helps people with Type 2 diabetes reduce heart disease risk. Here's how: The gel formed from soluble fiber traps substances in the intestinal tract that the body could eventually turn into fat and cholesterol; the gel is then passed from the body as part of the body's intestinal wastes. This process works exceptionally well when the intake of insoluble fiber is also high because the stools are heavier and pass through the intestinal tract much faster.

Overall, fiber may also help lower blood sugar levels. A study published in the prestigious *New England Journal of Medicine,* May 11, 2000, reported the effects of a high-fiber diet in adults with Type 2 diabetes. It compared the effects of two diets containing an equal number of calories but different amounts of fiber. During the first six weeks of the study, six participants ate a diet containing 50 grams of daily fiber, while seven others ate a diet containing 24 grams. Later, the participants switched diets. The researchers prepared all food. Compared with the low-fiber diet, the high-fiber diet reduced blood sugar levels and blood fats by 10 percent and reduced LDL cholesterol levels by 6 percent. The high-fiber diet also improved plasma insulin concentrations, dropping them by about 12 percent compared to people eating the lower fiber diet.

A Note About the Preventive Power of Carbohydrate-Rich Foods and Fiber

Researchers from the University of Minnesota and the Harvard School of Public Health studied 35,988 women in Iowa who were free of diabetes at the time of entry into the study. After six years, 1,141 women had developed Type 2 diabetes. Certain dietary factors were found to protect against the development of Type 2 diabetes— namely, the women who ate more whole grain fiber, cereal fiber, and dietary magnesium were less likely to develop diabetes.

Most strikingly, a diabetes expert commented in an editorial in the same issue of that journal, the benefits of the high-fiber diet for blood sugar levels are comparable to those seen when an antidiabetic drug is taken to lower blood sugar levels.

The researchers who conducted the study reported that there was no significant weight loss in either group, which told them that the improvement in blood sugars, plasma insulin concentration, and blood lipids was not due to caloric restriction (which is also known to improve all these factors).

The November 1997 issue of *Diabetes Care* reviewed the role of fiber, especially soluble fiber, as an aid in decreasing glucose absorption in the small intestine. The report indicated that including soluble fiber in a meal reduces the glycemic peak by an astonishing 50 percent. It also noted that soluble fiber causes a significant lowering of LDL cholesterol. How much soluble fiber? The researchers believe that people with Type 2 diabetes should take in about 3 grams of beta glucan. Two of the best sources of beta glucan soluble fiber are barley and oats. The best time to take such fiber is in the morning, to get the day off to a good start. We know that a lower glycemic response from one meal influences the glycemic response of the meals for the rest of the day. You will notice that I've included several recipes for oatmeal and breakfast barley as well as suggestions for several other ways to consume barley and oats throughout the day.

Similarly, the August 1997 issue of *Medical Hypotheses* reported that increasing soluble fiber is a valuable aid in blunting rapid blood sugar increases. This article suggests also that soluble fiber might correct the problems that occur in vascular smooth muscle (the muscle inside blood vessels), which eventually lead to microvascular complications.

There is absolutely no reason not to increase your fiber levels because we know with certainty that fiber is important in the overall strategy to lower blood cholesterol levels, especially LDL. For diabetics this action alone could be life-saving. Put another way, increasing the amount of soluble and insoluble fiber in your diet may be an important part of the dietary treatment of Type 2 diabetes—*of eating away your disease.*

Incidentally, we know from the National Center for Health Statistics that the vast majority of people with diabetes eat fewer than the 20 to 35 grams of fiber recommended daily by the American Diabetes Association.

The following table will help you plan your meals. It lists both the soluble and insoluble fiber in foods. Of course, the menus in Chapter Eight include plenty of these foods!

FIBER

Food Item	Amount	Grams of Total Fiber	Grams of Soluble Fiber
Corn	½ cup	1.6	0.1
Raw spinach	2 cups	1.6	0.4
Pumpernickel bread	1 piece	1.7	0.8
Strawberries	½ cup	1.8	0.6
Rye bread	1 piece	1.9	0.8
Broccoli	1 cup	2.1	0.2
Ground cinnamon	2 teaspoons	2.2	Not listed
Flaxseed	1 tablespoon	2.2	Not listed
Rye crisps	8 each	2.6	0.3
Kiwifruit	1 each	2.6	1.1
Banana	1 each	2.8	0.9
Dried coconut	¼ cup	3.2	0.3
Rye melba toast	8 each	3.2	0.7
Winter squash (acorn)	½ cup	3.2	0.3
Sun-dried tomatoes	½ cup	3.3	0.8
Asparagus	10 each	3.4	0.4
Banana chips	½ cup	3.5	0.97
Total wheat cereal	1 cup	3.5	2.4
Air-popped popcorn	3 cups	3.6	Not listed
Toasted wheat germ	¼ cup	3.6	0.2
Carrots	2 large	4.0	Not listed
Pear	1 each	4.0	0.8
Bulgur wheat, cooked	½ cup	4.1	0.7
Raspberries	½ cup	4.2	0.8

(continued)

Food Item	Amount	Grams of Total Fiber	Grams of Soluble Fiber
Dried apple rings	8 each	4.5	0.9
Grape-Nuts cereal	½ cup	4.6	2.5
Dried cranberries	½ cup	4.6	Not listed
Whole wheat pita pocket	1 each	4.7	2.1
Black-eyed peas, cooked	½ cup	5.6	0.7
Dried apricots	½ cup	5.8	3.4
Dried prunes	½ cup	6.0	2.5
Chickpeas, cooked	½ cup	6.2	1.94
Bran flakes cereal	1 cup	6.2	1.3
Shredded wheat and bran cereal	1 cup	6.3	Not listed
Spanish peanuts	½ cup	6.5	1.8
Dry-roasted pistachios	½ cup	6.6	0.2
Dried peaches	½ cup	6.6	2.6
Navy beans, canned	½ cup	6.7	4.01
Barley, cooked	½ cup	6.8	1.4
Lima beans, cooked	½ cup	7.0	1.9
Roasted soybeans	½ cup	7.0	3.0
Dry-roasted sunflower seeds	½ cup	7.1	2.3
Pinto beans, cooked	½ cup	7.4	2.7
Avocado	½ each	7.5	4.5
Black beans, cooked	½ cup	7.5	2.1
Raisin bran cereal	1 cup	7.7	2.0
Mung beans, cooked	½ cup	7.7	1.4
Lentils, cooked	½ cup	7.8	1.3
Black beans, cooked	½ cup	8.1	4.5
Split peas, cooked	½ cup	8.1	2.5
Red kidney beans, cooked	½ cup	8.2	6.3
Cooked spinach	2 cups	8.6	1.8
Blanched almonds	½ cup	9.3	0.3

(continued)

Food Item	Amount	Grams of Total Fiber	Grams of Soluble Fiber
Whole wheat bagel	1 each	10.3	3.9
Dry-roasted pecans	4 ounces	10.7	2.6
Dried figs	5 each	11.4	3.2
Rye wafers/crackers	8 each	20.1	4.64

What You Should Know About the Glycemic Index

The glycemic index is at best controversial in the scheme of what to do about taking care of your Type 2 diabetes, but there are a few things you should know about it.

> **Rather than choosing foods based on their glycemic index, it is better to choose a wide variety of carbohydrate-rich foods and ones that offer lots of fiber and a rich assortment of nutrients.**

Let's start with a look at the obvious factors that influence how your blood sugar responds to foods that contain carbohydrates. After consuming a particular carbohydrate-containing food, the rise in your blood sugar level depends on how many grams of carbohydrates are consumed; the percentage of the carbohydrates consumed that is absorbed by the small intestine; and the rate at which the carbohydrates are absorbed. Many different factors impact the rate of carbohydrate absorption, especially fiber.

Even when the same person consumes the same number of grams of carbohydrates at different times on an empty stomach, blood glucose levels respond differently. This is one reason that the glycemic index was developed. It measures the effect of specific carbohydrate-containing foods on the body's glucose levels.

In order to have a point of comparison, a standard food was chosen, and foods are compared to this standard food and given a value. The standard food is white bread, whose glycemic index is 100. To calculate the glycemic index, an amount of food with the same number of grams of carbohydrates is eaten alone, without any other foods. This is one of the criticisms of the glycemic index: When we eat a meal, we eat several foods, and each food greatly influences the glycemic index of other foods in that meal. In order to determine the glycemic index for any particular food, researchers measure the blood sugar response of ten people who are fed an equal amount of that food, and then calculate the average glycemic response.

Carbohydrate-rich foods have been categorized as being either high glycemic index foods, which means they cause a sharp, rapid increase in blood glucose levels when consumed alone, or low glycemic index foods, which cause a lower and steadier increase in blood glucose levels when consumed.

Some generalizations can be drawn about high glycemic foods versus low glycemic foods: More refined carbohydrates such as white bread, white bagels, white rice, and potatoes tend to be high glycemic index foods. Food with a higher fiber content and less refined carbohydrates tend to be low glycemic index foods; these include many fruits, vegetables, grains, and legumes. However, there are exceptions to this generalization.

Controversies nag at the usefulness of the glycemic index. The wide variety of factors that have an impact on the utility of the glycemic index include the following:

- Day-to-day variation: Glycemic responses can vary from day to day in the same person.

- Person-to-person variability: The same food in the same quantity can produce a very different glycemic response from one person to another.

- Carbohydrate-rich foods that one would think are healthier can have a higher glycemic index than a counterpart that seems less healthful. For example, Frosted Flakes has a glycemic index of 55, whereas fiber-rich Bran Flakes has a glycemic index of 74.

- All bets are off on the utility of the glycemic index in a mixed meal. For example, adding margarine or sour cream to a baked potato or eating the potato with a piece of meat can significantly change the glycemic index of the potato even though it remains the only carbohydrate-rich food in that meal. In a mixed meal the fat slows gastric emptying;

therefore, intestinal absorption is slowed, and then blood glucose rises much more slowly. This is why potato chips have a lower glycemic response than a baked potato—the potato chips are coated with fat. But who in their right nutrition mind would tell anyone to eat potato chips instead of a baked potato?

Probably the most important factor to decide whether or not the glycemic index should be used is that of individual variability. While glycemic index charts represent the average of many people, any one person cannot guess how he or she will respond to that food. You may have a high glycemic response to a food that generally has a low glycemic index, but have a low glycemic response to one that generally elicits a high glycemic response on average.

Glycemic Index Values of Common Foods

The chart given here is based on the averages obtained by many different studies conducted to determine the glycemic index for various food items.

Food Item	Glycemic Index Value
Apple	36
Apple juice	41
Apricots, dried	31
Bagel, white	72
Banana	53
Barley, pearled	25
Black-eyed beans	42
Bread, bulgur	52
Bread, mixed grain	45
Bread, oat bran	65
Bread, rye	56
Bread, wheat	70
Buckwheat	54

(continued)

Food Item	Glycemic Index Value
Bulgur	48
Bun, hamburger	61
Carrots	71
Cereal, All-Bran	42
Cereal, Bran Chex	58
Cereal, Cheerios	74
Cereal, Muesli	66
Cereal, Shredded Wheat	69
Cereal, Special K	54
Chickpeas	33
Chips, corn	73
Corn, sweet	55
Couscous	65
Cream of Wheat	66
Cream of Wheat, instant	74
Flour, whole meal	69
Honey	73
Ice cream	61
Kidney beans	27
Kiwifruit	52
Lentils, green	30
Mango	55
Melba toast	70
Milk, full fat	27
Oat bran, raw	55
Oatmeal	55
Orange	43
Orange juice	57
Pasta, white	41
Peach	28
Peanuts	14

(continued)

Food Item	Glycemic Index Value
Pear	36
Peas	48
Plum	64
Popcorn	55
Potato, baked	85
Potato, boiled	56
Potato, mashed	70
Raisins	65
Rice cakes	82
Rice, instant	91
Rock melon	65
Rye crisps	65
Soda crackers	72
Soft drink	68
Soybeans	18
Sweet potato	54
Watermelon	22
Yam	51
Yogurt, low fat, with artificial sweetener	14
Yogurt, low fat, fruited, sugar sweetened	33

Source: Nutrition Today, volume 34, number 2 (March/April 1999).

What You Should Know About Carbohydrates

You should now have a better understanding of carbohydrates. Remember the following important points:

- Carbohydrates are one type of energy found in food.
- Carbohydrates are the highest octane—the most desirable—fuel for the human body.

- For a person with Type 2 diabetes, approximately 50 to 60 percent of calories should come from carbohydrates.

- The carbohydrates you consume should come from carbohydrate-rich foods that are close to the form that occurs in nature. Some examples:

  - Whole grains and whole grain foods; a bulgur wheat pilaf is preferable to white bread;

  - Legumes, such as lentils, split peas, kidney beans, and black beans;

  - Whole fruits and vegetables; an apple is better than apple juice; a baked potato with skin is better than the flesh alone;

  - Nonfat and low-fat diary foods; skim milk is better than whole milk; low-fat and nonfat yogurt are better than whole milk yogurt.

Carbohydrates May Reduce the Rate of Progression of Type 2 Diabetes

Researchers from the University of Toronto studied ninety-one people with Type 2 diabetes. Some of them increased the carbohydrate content of their diet by using whole grain breakfast cereals, while others did not. After six months those who had increased their consumption of high-fiber carbohydrates by eating breakfast cereal showed no change in glycemic control (i.e., their mean blood sugar levels did not change), but they did have significantly fewer free fatty acids. The researchers say that this reduction in free fatty acids associated with higher carbohydrate intake may reduce the rate of progression of Type 2 diabetes.

- Increasing the fiber content of your diet helps to reduce the risk of heart disease and may help moderate rises in blood sugar.

- Until proven otherwise, it is not worth modifying your diet to accommodate the glycemic index. Instead, focus on the factors recommended above.

Chapter Five

Why Your Choice of Protein Foods Matters

Protein may be shrouded in as many misconceptions as carbohydrates. Probably the most common *and dangerous* misconception is that high-protein diets can help control diabetes.

If you follow one of the new high-protein diets, you will miss out on many nutrients you need for good health and for better control of your blood sugars. Limiting carbohydrate-containing foods is downright danger-ous for you. Meals too low in carbohydrates cause the body to produce high levels of free fatty acids, and *free fatty acids are dangerous for people with diabetes*. They cause insulin resistance and the resultant bad effects on heart health and health in general.

This isn't to say that you don't need protein; indeed, protein is an essen-tial nutrient for good health.

As a diabetic, you need to realize that your health profile
will improve substantially when you choose
protein foods carefully.

Believe it or not, your choice of protein foods significantly influences your risk of coronary artery disease. You therefore need to understand how to make choices that will improve your health overall.

What Is Protein, and What Is Its Role in Good Health?

Just as there are carbohydrates and carbohydrate-containing foods, the same is true for protein. There is the macronutrient protein, and there are protein-containing foods.

Let's take a look first at protein as the nutrient it is.

Protein is a calorie-containing nutrient with another job. In Chapter 4 Four you learned that there are three types of calorie-containing nutrients: carbohydrates, proteins, and fat. Indeed, protein supplies calories to the body. Like carbohydrates, protein supplies about 4 calories per gram. A 2-ounce piece of salmon, for example, has about 14 grams of protein, which accounts for about 58 of the 100 calories in that portion. (The remainder of the calories come from fat, much of it a healthier fat called omega-3, which you will learn about in Chapter Six.)

But protein has even more important roles than supplying calories to the body. The following are the vital roles that protein plays in our health:

- Protein is the most important nutrient for supporting growth and tissue repair; it is at work in every cell of the body.

- Protein-rich substances drive the body's never-ending chemical reactions that make us breathe, keep our heart beating, and stimulate every other action vital to life.

- Without protein our hormones, antibodies (essential to fighting infections), and genes (the body's code for making any tissue or cell) could not function.

- Protein substances maintain the optimal chemical mixture in the blood for good health.

It is no wonder, then, that the word *protein* comes from the Greek *proteios,* which means holding first place.

A microscopic look at proteins.   Proteins are constructed of building blocks called amino acids. Like carbohydrates and fats, amino acids are made of carbon, hydrogen, and oxygen molecules. But an additional element, nitrogen, distinguishes proteins from these other energy sources.

Amino acids are joined together in thousands of ways to form long chains called peptides. Two proteins that have totally different functions—liver protein and muscle protein, for example—can be composed of exactly the same amino acids. The difference lies in how the amino acids are linked together.

There are two categories of amino acids: essential and nonessential. These categories have nothing to do with how important each is in the body. Rather, they distinguish the amino acids the body can make from those it cannot. Of the twenty-two amino acids needed, nine are dietary *essentials,* or must be obtained through the diet. The remaining thirteen are *nonessential* because the body can make them from scraps of leftover carbohydrates, fats, and other amino acids.

Why essential amino acids are . . . so essential. If you lack just one essential amino acid for any period of time—no matter how many other amino acids you consume—your body will break down your own muscle tissue to harvest that essential amino acid. This is because your body needs to build hormones and perform functions less vital than building and maintaining muscle tissue.

The reason we don't worry much about adequate protein intake in the United States is that Americans generally eat too much protein. About 16 percent of their calories comes from protein, when only about 10 percent is required for optimal health. So most of us eat far too much protein.

Let's take a look at why essential amino acids are essential. If you get all your protein from plant sources, you may not be taking in all the essential amino acids in a day's time. While animal and marine proteins—eggs, cheese, milk, meat, chicken, and fish—contain all essential amino acids, most plant proteins do not. Soybeans and foods made from soybeans, as well as some nuts, are said to be "weakly complete," which means they contain all essential amino acids but have relatively small amounts of one or more of them, making it difficult to assemble body proteins.

Fortunately, though, with just a little dietary maneuvering, weakly complete and even incomplete proteins can be used to supply the body with all essential amino acids. To do this we simply "complement" one incomplete protein food with another one; that is, we eat foods that have different complements of amino acids. The sidebar entitled Complementing Incomplete Proteins will help you make these combinations. It's really quite easy.

The good news is that you only have to have a complement of complete proteins over the course of a full day's time. For many years nutrition experts thought that incomplete proteins had to be complemented in the same meal to ensure their use as protein instead of fuel. (That is what happens to leftover essential amino acids—they get recycled as fuel, and not even the best type of fuel, as we will see below.) Now we know, however, that incomplete protein foods need only be complemented within a day's time. We also know that having a very small quantity of a complete protein food with an incomplete one—such as a bit of cheese with beans and rice— also ensures that the protein in the incomplete protein food will hook up with the other essential amino acids it needs to make a complete protein.

Steering yourself toward vegetarian eating.   Some of you may be wondering why we're discussing plant sources of protein, or "vegetarian eating." Maybe you are a confirmed meat eater. You may be thinking that vegetarian main courses will never touch your lips. It is my intention to help you, gently but firmly, modify your thinking. If it's hard to stomach the concept of vegetarian eating (sorry for the play on words), then just think about including more plant sources of protein.

Including more plant sources of protein is another way to eat away Type 2 diabetes and the associated risk of artery-clogging heart disease (atherosclerosis).

If nothing else, think of your pocketbook: Eating more plant sources of protein is a great way to eat for far less money. In addition, the recipes in this book will get you started on fabulously great meals that just don't happen to have any meat.

Why Protein Isn't the Best Energy Source

Here is an analogy to make the point. Many people heat their homes with natural gas. While some by-products result from the process of burning natural

Complementing Incomplete Proteins

For those of you who want to try more plant sources of protein, here is a list that will help you complement your proteins—or make sure you get all essential amino acids in a day's time. There is one easy rule to keep in mind: Eat grain foods with legumes. The following combinations of foods give you all essential amino acids:

- Lentils and corn (such as lentil soup and corn bread)
- Rice and kidney beans
- Tofu (or other forms of soy) and rice
- Peanut butter and whole wheat bread
- Corn tortilla and pinto beans
- Meatless chili with beans and whole wheat bread
- Navy beans and rye bread
- Rice cakes and peanut butter
- Chickpeas and corn bread
- Black-eyed peas and corn bread

Don't forget, though, that if you have one source of complete protein during the day, such as a glass of skim milk, some yogurt, or a piece of fish, you will have accomplished this task without having to worry about complementing incomplete sources of protein.

gas, there are relatively few—especially compared with the outrageous alternative of burning a varnished mahogany dining room table to heat your home. Burning the table would produce heat but at great cost, and not just the financial loss of a family antique. There would also be the nasty by-products released when the stain and varnish burn.

As outrageous as this example seems, it is somewhat akin to relying on protein as your main source of calories, as would be the case if you went on one of those fad high-protein diets. The unwanted by-products of burning protein for energy—ketones among them—must pass through the kidneys to be excreted through the urine. While many people can handle the process of getting rid of all these unwanted by-products, others cannot, and people with Type 2 diabetes might be among those who cannot.

In addition, if you rely on protein as your main source of calories, you would get more than you bargained for. If you eat meat, chicken, or eggs as part of this protein, then you get far too much fat and cholesterol. As a person with diabetes, this extra fat and cholesterol has the potential of increasing your risk for atherosclerosis, which is already accelerated by virtue of the fact that you have diabetes.

How Much Protein Do You Need Daily?

Much less than most of us eat! For the majority of Americans, protein may well be the most overconsumed nutrient. We are a land of plenty, where plenty means 20-ounce steaks and double burgers. Let's run through a few numbers to help you understand your protein needs.

Before continuing, I must add this caveat: If you have any type of kidney disease from Type 2 diabetes or any other reason, your protein needs might be considerably different. Please ask your physician if your protein needs are different from the recommended amounts for most Americans.

Every day each of us needs about .8 gram of protein for every kilogram of body weight. This may sound like Greek to you, so here is a translation:

One kilogram of body weight equals 2.2 pounds.

To determine body weight in kilograms, divide the body weight in pounds by 2.2. For example, a person who weighs 150 pounds weighs about 68 kilograms.

To determine protein needs, multiply 68 kilograms by .8 gram of protein per kilogram: $68 \times .8 = 54$ grams of protein.

You may think this sounds like too little protein because most Americans eat closer to 100 grams daily, and many eat much more than that.

More Reasons to Avoid High-Protein Diets

While high-protein diets aren't a healthy alternative for anyone, here are the reasons that you, a person with diabetes, should run, not walk, as far away from them as you can:

- The extra protein is a strain on your kidneys (as it is for infants, children, and adults with kidney failure from other causes).
- When high-protein diets also restrict carbohydrates severely, they create a metabolic state that can stress the kidneys and cause the body to break down muscle.
- Studies have not shown an association between protein intake and leanness. Lean people don't consume more protein than overweight people. In fact, heavier people generally consume more protein than lean people.
- A meat-centered, high-fat diet with too few fruits or vegetables promotes both weight gain and heart disease.

DOES A HIGH-PROTEIN DIET INCREASE MUSCLE MASS?

Many people ask if eating more protein can help them build more muscle or lean body tissue. There is no evidence to indicate that you can increase muscle mass, or "bulk up," by eating more protein. In fact, exercise experts have shown in repeated studies that people who work out may need *less* protein than those who do not. This is because exercising regularly helps the body retain nitrogen, one of the building blocks of protein. The best and only way to build more muscle tissue is to use your muscles. Yes, "use it or lose it" is true here! Use your muscle tissue every single day, as much as you can, and you will not only retain it but also build more. As you will learn in Chapter Seven, this is extremely important for a person with diabetes or at risk of diabetes.

A simpler way of determining protein needs. The American Diabetes Association, along with other major health organizations in this country, recommends that people with diabetes get about 10 to 20 percent of their calories from protein. The meal plans in this book follow these guidelines.

Do Protein Needs Change Because You Have Diabetes?

As noted above, your protein needs may be lower if you have damage to your kidneys. That is why it is important to ask your physician about your kidneys before you follow the meal plans in this book.

There is one other factor about protein needs in people with diabetes. Clinical research has shown that those whose diabetes is not well controlled—in other words, their blood sugars are ranging out of control—may burn up their muscle tissue. Rather than eat more protein, you should instead work hard to bring your blood sugars under control.

What Kind of Protein Should You Eat?

You have reached the most important part of this chapter—the part that tells you what type of protein to eat!

Choosing your protein foods optimally is one way to eat away your diabetes and also slash your heightened risk of heart disease.

Here are the guidelines for you, a person with diabetes and therefore a person with a heightened risk of heart disease. These guidelines are also fabulous for people who don't have a disease, but they are essential for you to follow. After you look at these guidelines, keep reading to learn the huge differences in the overall nutritional value of different types of protein.

- *Breakfast protein:* Choose from the following sources of protein:
  —Egg whites
  —Nonfat liquid egg substitute
  —Tofu (you'll find some great recipes for smoothies and tofu scrambles)
  —Skim milk or reduced fat and fortified soy milk
  —Nonfat cottage cheese
  —Bacon or sausage made from soy products

- *Lunch protein:* Your meals should consist almost entirely of two types of protein:
  —The main source should be from vegetables (such as black beans and lentils), nuts, and fish (canned is okay).
  —Most of your meals should also contain either skim milk or soy milk.
  —It's okay to have a lean meat sandwich or a cheese-containing dish once or twice a week at lunch; in fact, these meals have been built into the thirty days of good eating planned for you.

- *Dinner protein:* Think of this protein in seven-day cycles. In each cycle, I'd like you to plan:
  —at least two fish meals, though more is better (and canned is okay);
  —at least two vegetable sources of protein, though more is better; and
  —one of the following for the other three days:
    - two poultry meals and one red meat meal (red meat is beef, pork, veal, lamb, and game meat). Of course, you don't have to have these meals; it is perfectly okay—and even better—to substitute more fish or more vegetable sources of protein.
    - two red meat meals and one poultry meal. Remember, you can take away any of these and have more fish or vegetable sources of protein.

Take a look at the following chart that gives an example of one way to divide up your dinner protein. Each of the items listed is intended as an entrée. Recipes for each of the items here are in Chapter Twelve.

Monday	Tuesday	Wednesday	Thursday	Friday	Saturday	Sunday
Foiled Salmon and Veggies	Grilled Beef Fajitas	Black Bean Soup with Cilantro	Crab à la Tuna Cakes	Tomato-Barley Chicken Stew	Sage-Simmered Pork Chops	"Lobster" with Basil-Caper Drizzle
Barbeque Meat Loaf	Southwest Tuna and Salsa	Oven-Fried Chicken	Fresh Vegetable and Lentil Salad	Lemon-Fresh Salmon Loaf	Cream of Mushroom and Barley Soup	Checker-board Baked Beans
White Bean and Tomato Pasta Sauce	Pork Tenderloin Stir-Fry	Black Bean and Artichoke Pita	Lemon Pepper Sizzled Tilapia	Sesame Ginger Chicken Stir-Fry	Classic Spaghetti	Ginger-Seared Sole
Creamy Chicken and Rice	Cream of Asparagus Soup	Lemon-and-Orange-Roasted Red Snapper	Herbed Chicken and Pasta	Lentil Stew	Pineapple Salmon	Beef Stew

A note about portion sizes: As mentioned above, it is the rare American who consumes too little protein. One of the main reasons is that our protein portions are far too large. While you should buy a food scale to weigh your protein portions, here are some visuals to help you understand the optimal protein food sizes:

- For meat and poultry, a good serving size is 3 cooked ounces, which is about the size of a deck of playing cards in height, width, and thickness.
  —To create another visual, envision a 1-pound package of ground sirloin. A package this size should serve four people.
  —Yet another visual: Recall what two chicken thighs look like; this would be an optimal portion size for one person.

- For fish, plan on 3 to 5 ounces, depending on what you are eating the rest of the day. Why can you have more fish than meat or poultry? Because the calories per ounce are a lot fewer, and some fish has the added bonus of omega-3 fatty acids, which can be a help in reducing your risk of heart disease.

- For beans, such as black beans and lentils, a good portion size is about one cup after cooking.

- For tofu, an optimal portion size is about 6 ounces of light (alias for "reduced-fat") tofu, which is about one-half of one of those cardboard boxes. For tempeh, about 3 ounces.

- Cheese is a difficult one because a healthy size is so tiny unless you switch to 50% reduced-fat or soy cheese.

  —Shredded cheese: ¼ cup, which is the equivalent of 1 ounce, and I insist you measure it with a measuring cup.

  —Sliced cheese: Generally one slice (this is a great way to practice portion control).

  —Cheese from a block: 1 ounce, which is somewhat equivalent to the size of a pair of dice.

More on Why Choice of Protein Matters

I've compiled an interesting set of facts here. Included is information about how much of the following high-protein foods is needed to yield 14 grams of protein, which is about the amount of protein found in 2 ounces of most meat and poultry. Then, I've tallied certain facts that should be very revealing for you, and will help you understand why it is so important for your good health to choose some vegetable and fish sources of protein instead of all meat. Following this chart are calculations to prove this point from another point of view and to ensure that you realize how important this all is!

BEEF (PER 14 GRAMS PROTEIN)

	Calories	Fat Grams	% Fat Calories	Saturated Fat Grams	% of Calories as Saturated Fat	Fiber Grams	Omega-3 Fat Grams	Bonus Nutrients*
Regular hamburger, 22% fat (1¾ ounces)	157	10.7	63	4.2	25	0	0.04	
Lean hamburger, 16% fat (2 ounces)	142	9.2	60	3.6	23	0	0.04	Riboflavin (8%), Niacin (12%), B₁₂ (16%), Selenium (15%), Zinc (20%)
Beef sirloin (1¾ ounces)	112	6.0	50	2.3	19	0	0.05	Niacin (9%), B₆ (9%), B₁₂ (23%), Iron (8%), Phosphorus (11%), Selenium (19%), Zinc (22%)
Beef tenderloin (2 ounces)	194	15.1	71	6.0	28	0	0.14	Riboflavin (9%), Niacin (9%), B₆ (9%), B₁₂ (24%), Iron (10%), Phosphorus (12%), Selenium (19%), Zinc (17%)
Beef eye of round roast (1¾ ounces)	85	2.7	30	1.0	11	0	0	Niacin (9%), B₆ (9%), B₁₂ (18%), Phosphorus (11%), Selenium (19%), Zinc (16%)
Beef rib eye steak (2 ounces)	174	12.6	67	5.1	27	0	0	Niacin (12%), B₆ (10%), B₁₂ (28%), Phosphorus (10%), Selenium (18%), Zinc (23%)

*At 8% or Greater of the Daily Value

PORK (PER 14 GRAMS PROTEIN)

	Calories	Fat Grams	% Fat Calories	Saturated Fat Grams	% of Calories as Saturated Fat	Fiber Grams	Omega-3 Fat Grams	Bonus Nutrients*
Tenderloin (1¾ ounces)	100	4.0	38	1.5	14	0	0.01	Thiamin (32%), Riboflavin (11%), Niacin (13%), B$_6$ (13%), B$_{12}$ (8%), Phosphorus (14%), Selenium (34%), Zinc (10%)
Pork chop, sirloin, boneless (1¾ ounces)	87	3.3	35	1.2	13	0	0	Thiamin (23%), Riboflavin (8%), Niacin (10%), B$_6$ (11%), Phosphorus (9%), Selenium (30%), Zinc (8%)

*At 8% or Greater of the Daily Value

POULTRY (PER 14 GRAMS PROTEIN)

	Calories	Fat Grams	% Fat Calories	Saturated Fat Grams	% of Calories as Saturated Fat	Fiber Grams	Omega-3 Fat Grams	Bonus Nutrients*
Chicken breast, boneless, roasted, served with skin (1¾ ounces)	98	3.9	37	1.1	10	0	0.05	Niacin (32%), B$_6$ (14%), Phosphorus (11%), Selenium (18%)
Chicken breast, batter fried (2 ounces)	147	7.5	47	2.0	12	0.2	0.1	Niacin (30%), B$_6$ (12%), Phosphorus (10%), Selenium (23%)

(continued)

POULTRY *(cont.)*	Calories	Fat Grams	% Fat Calories	Saturated Fat Grams	% of Calories as Saturated Fat	Fiber Grams	Omega-3 Fat Grams	Bonus Nutrients*
Fried chicken wing, with skin (2 ounces)	182	12.6	64	3.4	17	0.1	0.2	
Breaded chicken, with skin (2½ ounces)	206	12.8	57	3.4	15	0.4	0.2	Riboflavin (12%), Niacin (17%), B₆ (8%), Pantothenic Acid (12%), Phosphorus (11%), Selenium (24%), Zinc (10%)
Baked chicken, skin removed after baking (2½ ounces)	69	0.4	5	0.1	1	0	0	Copper (9%), Phosphorus (20%)
Turkey breast, boneless, skinless (1¾ ounces)	67	0.4	5	0.1	2	0	0	Niacin (19%), B₆ (14%), Phosphorus (11%), Selenium (23%)
Turkey, dark meat, boneless, skinless (1¾ ounces)	80	2.1	25	0.7	8	0	0.03	Niacin (9%), B₆ (9%), Phosphorus (10%), Selenium (29%), Zinc (14%)
Turkey, white and dark meat, skinless (1¾ ounces)	84	2.5	28	0.8	9	0	0.04	Niacin (14%), B₆ (11%), Phosphorus (11%), Selenium (26%), Zinc (10%)
Turkey with skin	94	3.7	37	1.0	10	0	0.05	

*At 8% or Greater of the Daily Value

FISH (PER 14 GRAMS PROTEIN)

	Calories	Fat Grams	% Fat Calories	Saturated Fat Grams	% of Calories as Saturated Fat	Fiber Grams	Omega-3 Fat Grams	Bonus Nutrients*
Tuna (white or Albacore), packed in water (2 ounces)	73	1.7	22	0.5	6	0	0.53	Niacin (16%), B$_{12}$ (11%), Vitamin D (23%), Phosphorus (12%), Selenium (53%)
Tuna (white or Albacore), packed in oil, drained (1¾ ounces)	92	4	41	0.8	8	0	0.5	Niacin (29%), B$_6$ (11%), B$_{12}$ (18%), Vitamin D (25%), Phosphorus (13%), Selenium (43%)
Tuna (light), packed in water, drained (2 ounces)	66	0.5	7	0.1	2	0	0.15	Niacin (38%), B$_6$ (10%), B$_{12}$ (28%), Vitamin D (23%), Phosphorus (9%), Selenium (65%)
Pink salmon, canned in water with bones, not drained (2½ ounces)	99	4.3	41	1.1	10	0	1.2	Riboflavin (8%), Niacin (23%), B$_6$ (11%), B$_{12}$ (52%), Vitamin D (111%), Calcium (15%), Phosphorus (23%), Selenium (34%)
Baked wild salmon (2 ounces)	103	4.6	42	0.7	6	0	1.3	Thiamin (10%), Riboflavin (16%), Niacin (29%), B$_6$ (27%), B$_{12}$ (29%), Vitamin D (40%), Pantothenic Acid (11%), Phosphorus (15%), Potassium (10%), Selenium (38%)

(continued)

83

FISH (cont.)	Calories	Fat Grams	% Fat Calories	Saturated Fat Grams	% of Calories as Saturated Fat	Fiber Grams	Omega-3 Fat Grams	Bonus Nutrients*
Tuna steak (1¾ ounces)	65	0.6	9	0.2	3	0	0.2	Niacin (47%), B_6 (24%), B_{12} (18%), Phosphorus (14%), Selenium (33%)
Canned mackerel (2 ounces)	88	3.6	38	1.1	11	0	0.72	Niacin (18%), B_{12} (66%), Vitamin D (64%), Calcium (14%), Phosphorus (17%), Selenium (31%)
Anchovies, canned in oil, drained (1¼ ounces)	104	1.1	43	1.1	10	0	1.03	Riboflavin (11%), Niacin (49%), B_{12} (7%), Vitamin E (12%), Calcium (12%), Iron (13%), Copper (8%), Magnesium (9%), Phosphorus (13%), Potassium (8%), Selenium (48%), Zinc (8%)
Lake trout (2¼ ounces)	85	3.0	33	0.8	9	0	0.3	Riboflavin (8%), Niacin (9%), B_6 (15%), B_{12} (37%), Phosphorus (20%), Potassium (8%), Selenium (43%)
Catfish, broiled (2½ ounces)	120	6.7	52	1.6	12	0	0	Thiamin (17%), Niacin (9%), B_6 (7%), B_{12} (31%), Vitamin D (89%), Pantothenic Acid (7%), Phosphorus (16%)
Snapper (2 ounces)	73	1.0	13	0.2	3	0	0.2	B_6 (13%), B_{12} (33%), Phosphorus (11%), Potassium (8%), Selenium (40%)

	Calories	Fat Grams	% Fat Calories	Saturated Fat Grams	% of Calories as Saturated Fat	Fiber Grams		Bonus Nutrients*
Flounder/sole (2 ounces)	66	0.9	12	0.2	3	0	0.3	B_{12} (24%), Vitamin D (9%), Magnesium (8%), Phosphorus (16%), Selenium (47%)
Sea bass (2 ounces)	70	1.5	20	0.4	5	0	0.4	B_6 (13%), Magnesium (8%), Phosphorus (14%), Selenium (38%)
Cod (2½ ounces)	67	0.6	8	0.1	2	0	0.1	Niacin (8%), B_6 (9%), B_{12} (11%), Vitamin D (9%), Phosphorus (9%), Selenium (34%)
Halibut (2 ounces)	79	1.7	20	0.2	3	0	0.3	Niacin (20%), B_6 (11%), B_{12} (13%), Magnesium (15%), Phosphorus (16%), Potassium (9%), Selenium (38%)

*At 8% or Greater of the Daily Value

LEGUMES (PER 14 GRAMS PROTEIN)

	Calories	Fat Grams	% Fat Calories	Saturated Fat Grams	% of Calories as Saturated Fat	Fiber Grams	Bonus Nutrients*
Black beans (1 cup)	220	2	9	0	0	14	Thiamin (28%), Folate (64%), Copper (18%), Iron (20%), Magnesium (30%), Manganese (38%), Phosphorus (24%), Potassium (17%), Zinc (13%)
Lentils (¾ cup)	172	0.6	3	0.1	0	11.7	Thiamin (17%), Niacin (8%), B_6 (13%), Folate (67%), Copper (19%), Iron (27%), Magnesium (13%), Manganese (37%), Phosphorus (27%), Potassium (16%), Zinc (13%)

(continued)

85

LEGUMES (cont.)	Calories	Fat Grams	% Fat Calories	Saturated Fat Grams	% of Calories as Saturated Fat	Fiber Grams	Bonus Nutrients*
Kidney beans (1 cup)	225	0.9	3	0.1	0	11.3	Thiamin (19%), B$_6$ (11%), Folate (57%), Copper (21%), Iron (29%), Magnesium (20%), Manganese (42%), Phosphorus (25%), Potassium (20%), Zinc (13%)
White kidney beans (1¼ cups)	288	1.6	5				Thiamin (19%), Riboflavin (12%), Calcium (48%), Iron (31%), Phosphorus (39%)
Extra-firm lean tofu (7 ounces)	75	1.4	16	0.2	3	0	Folate (9%), Calcium (15%), Copper (13%), Iron (13%), Magnesium (25%), Manganese (67%), Phosphorus (23%), Selenium (23%), Zinc (11%)
Tempeh (2¾ ounces)	154	8.9	48	2.6	14		Riboflavin (16%), Niacin (8%), B$_6$ (8%), Copper (21%), Iron (9%), Magnesium (15%), Manganese (50%), Phosphorus (20%), Potassium (9%), Zinc (8%)
Green soy beans (4 ounces)	160	7.3	38	0.8	4	4.8	Thiamin (20%), Riboflavin (10%), Vitamin C (32%), Folate (31%), Calcium (16%), Iron (16%), Magnesium (17%), Manganese (28%), Phosphorus (18%), Potassium (17%)
Soy nuts (1½ ounces)	200	10.8	45	1.6	7	7.5	Folate (22%), Copper (18%), Iron (9%), Magnesium (15%), Manganese (46%), Phosphorus (15%), Potassium (18%), Selenium (12%), Zinc (9%)

	Calories	Fat Grams	% Fat Calories	Saturated Fat Grams	Fiber Grams		Bonus Nutrients*
Black-eyed peas (6 ounces)	197	0.9	4	0.2	1	11.1	Thiamin (23%), B$_6$ (9%), Folate (88%), Pantothenic Acid (8%), Copper (23%), Iron (24%), Magnesium (23%), Manganese (40%), Phosphorus (27%), Potassium (14%), Zinc (15%)
Pinto beans (6 ounces)	233	0.9	3	0.2	1	14.6	Thiamin (21%), Riboflavin (9%), B$_6$ (13%), Vitamin E (8%), Folate (73%), Calcium (8%), Copper (22%), Iron (25%), Magnesium (23%), Manganese (47%), Phosphorus (27%), Potassium (23%), Selenium (17%), Zinc (12%)

At 8% or Greater of the Daily Value

DAIRY (PER 14 GRAMS PROTEIN)

	Calories	Fat Grams	% Fat Calories	Saturated Fat Grams	Fiber Grams	Bonus Nutrients*
Skim milk (15 ounces)	148	0.8	5	0.5	0	Vitamin A (26%), Thiamin (10%), Riboflavin (35%), B$_6$ (9%), B$_{12}$ (27%), Vitamin D (43%), Pantothenic Acid (14%), Calcium (52%), Magnesium (12%), Phosphorus (43%), Potassium (20%), Selenium (13%), Zinc (11%)
1% milk (15 ounces)	178	4.5	23	2.8	0	Vitamin A (25%), Thiamin (11%), Riboflavin (42%), B$_6$ (9%), B$_{12}$ (26%), Vitamin D (43%), Pantothenic Acid (14%), Calcium (52%), Magnesium (15%), Phosphorus (41%), Potassium (19%), Selenium (13%), Zinc (11%)
2% milk (15 ounces)	211	8.2	35	5.1	0	Vitamin A (24%), Thiamin (11%), Riboflavin (41%), B$_6$ (9%), B$_{12}$ (26%), Vitamin D (43%), Pantothenic Acid (14%), Calcium (52%), Magnesium (15%), Phosphorus (40%), Potassium (19%), Selenium (13%), Zinc (11%)

(continued)

DAIRY (cont.)	Calories	Fat Grams	% Fat Calories	Saturated Fat Grams	Fiber Grams	Bonus Nutrients*
Whole milk (15 ounces)	261	14.2	49	8.8	0	Vitamin A (13%), Thiamin (11%), Riboflavin (41%), B_6 (9%), B_{12} (25%), Vitamin D (43%), Pantothenic Acid (13%), Calcium (51%), Magnesium (14%), Phosphorus (40%), Potassium (18%), Selenium (12%), Zinc (11%)
Nonfat yogurt, plain (12 ounces)	150	0	0	0	0	Thiamin (8%), Riboflavin (34%), Vitamin B_{12} (25%), Pantothenic Acid (16%), Calcium (49%), Magnesium (12%), Phosphorus (38%), Potassium (18%), Selenium (13%), Zinc (16%)
Low-fat yogurt, plain (10 ounces)	179	4.4	22	2.8	0	Thiamin (8%), Riboflavin (36%), B_6 (7%), B_{12} (27%), Folate (8%), Pantothenic Acid (17%), Calcium (52%), Magnesium (12%), Phosphorus (41%), Potassium (19%), Selenium (13%), Zinc (17%)
Whole milk yogurt, plain (14 ounces)	244	12.9	47	8.3	0	Vitamin A (12%), Thiamin (8%), Riboflavin (33%), B_{12} (25%), Folate (7%), Pantothenic Acid (15%), Calcium (48%), Magnesium (11%), Phosphorus (38%), Potassium (18%), Selenium (12%), Zinc (16%)
Cheddar cheese (2 ounces)	228	18.8	74	12.0	0	Vitamin A (16%), Riboflavin (13%), B_{12} (8%), Calcium (41%), Phosphorus (29%), Selenium (11%), Zinc (12%)
50% reduced-fat cheddar cheese (1¾ ounces)	123	7.0	50	5.3	0	Vitamin A (15%), Calcium (35%)
Fat-free cheddar cheese (1¾ ounces)	71	0	0	0	0	Vitamin A (15%), Calcium (71%)

Food						At 8% or Greater of the Daily Value*
Mozzarella cheese (2½ ounces)	199	15.3	69	9.3	0	Vitamin A (17%), Riboflavin (10%), B_{12} (8%), Calcium (37%), Phosphorus (26%), Selenium (15%), Zinc (10%)
Part-skim mozzarella cheese (2 ounces)	144	9.0	57	5.7	0	Vitamin A (10%), Riboflavin (10%), B_{12} (8%), Calcium (37%), Phosphorus (26%), Selenium (12%), Zinc (10%)
Low-fat mozzarella cheese (1¾ ounces)	128	8.0	54	4.8	0	Vitamin A (9%), Riboflavin (10%), B_{12} (10%), Calcium (40%), Phosphorus (32%), Zinc (13%)
Whole egg (2)	149	10	62	3	0	Vitamin A (19%), Riboflavin (30%), B_{12} (17%), Vitamin D (13%), Folate (12%), Pantothenic Acid (13%), Iron (8%), Phosphorus (18%), Selenium (44%)
Egg white (4)	67	0	0	0	0	Riboflavin (36%), Selenium (34%)
Egg substitute (½ cup)	105	4.2	37	0.8	0	Vitamin A (27%), Riboflavin (22%), Vitamin D (12%), Pantothenic Acid (34%), Iron (15%), Phosphorus (15%), Potassium (12%), Selenium (45%), Zinc (11%)

At 8% or Greater of the Daily Value

What Do All These Charts Mean?

You have probably made some discoveries of your own after reading these charts, but here is what I hoped you would discover:

- High-protein foods with less fat give 14 grams of protein for far fewer calories.
- High-protein foods with less fat give many more bonus nutrients.
- Fish sources of protein give more bonuses than meat sources of protein; in addition, they give the same amount of protein for far fewer calories and rich amounts of protein for the bonus of omega-3 fatty acids, the wonderful fat that may help fight heart disease.
- Vegetable sources of protein, as compared to meat sources of protein, give several additional bonuses: fiber (which is not found in animal sources of protein), a higher percentage of bonus nutrients, negligible fat, and no saturated fat.

Now you know why I've highlighted certain choices in the chart. These are the ones I want you to concentrate on for getting your protein—the choices I encourage you to make.

One More Set of Calculations for You to Digest

As you know by now, I like you to have the maximum amount of information, so that you understand why I am encouraging you to make certain choices in protein foods. Here, I've tallied the results of serving certain types of protein food each night for one week:

Example #1: One Week's Worth of Dinner Protein
- 3 ounces broiled rib eye steak
- 3 ounces ground beef
- 3 ounces pork chop
- 3 ounces fried chicken breast
- 3 ounces sirloin steak

- 3 ounces chicken legs
- 3 ounces Kielbasa (sausage)

The tally for this week's worth of protein foods:

    1,564 calories

    143 grams protein

    0.26 grams fiber

    60 percent of calories as fat

    101 total grams fat

    36 grams saturated fat

Example #2: One Week's Worth of Dinner Protein

- 3 ounces broiled beef tenderloin
- 3 ounces baked or broiled salmon
- 3 ounces tuna in water
- 3 ounces roasted chicken breast
- ¾ cup lentils on a salad or in soup
- ½ cup black beans on a salad, in a soup, or as a tortilla
- Spaghetti made with half lean hamburger (1.5 ounces) and half vegetable ground round (1.5 ounces)

The tally for this week's worth of protein foods:

    1,032 calories

    133 grams protein

    21 grams fiber

    26 percent of calories as fat

    30 total grams fat

    9.3 grams saturated fat

What a difference!

It is hoped that you will be convinced to start making these changes and not balk at the vegetable sources of protein offered in the menu and recipe chapters.

What You've Learned About Protein Foods

Here is what you should have learned from this chapter:

- Pass up high-protein diets.
- Set your sites on taking in about 10 to 20 percent of your calories as protein.
- If your kidneys are damaged from diabetes, ask your doctor how much protein you should eat.
- Diversify your choices of dinner protein foods like this:
  —Have at least two fish meals weekly (more is better).
  —Have at least two vegetable sources of protein weekly (more is better).
  —For the remainder of your dinners, choose one lean skinless poultry meal and two lean beef meals, or vice versa.
- Have vegetable sources of protein for lunch as much as possible.
- When choosing meat and poultry, limit your portion to about 3 ounces, the size of a deck of playing cards. Because fish has many fewer calories and the bonus of omega-3 fats, you can go up to 5 ounces (again, as long as you don't have kidney problems that necessitate limiting your protein grams).

Chapter Six

Choose Your Fats Carefully

The word *fat* suffers from an instantly bad reputation. Whether we are referring to fat in food or fat on our body, most of us have this instant aversion to the word.

How Americans choose the amount of fats in their foods, however, is truly contrary to how they feel about the substance. Indeed, most Americans eat far more fat than is recommended by the American Heart Association, the American Diabetes Association, and the American Cancer Society.

As a person with diabetes, you have two huge reasons to care about fat intake:

1. Eating too much fat, especially saturated fat, will increase your risk of heart disease. As you've read in this book, heart disease is already a huge concern for you as a diabetic. There is also some evidence that excessive saturated fat can make it more difficult to control your diabetes.

2. Eating too much fat of any type makes it easier to gain weight and harder to bring weight down. You will learn more about this as you read on. You have already read that living at a weight higher than what is recommended for your height worsens your diabetes.

You should follow certain important guidelines in regard to fat intake:

- Decrease total fat calories per day to 30 percent or less of total calorie intake. (Note: People with excessively high triglyceride levels may need to raise dietary fat intake but only a specific type of dietary fat—monounsaturated fat.)

- Substitute better types of fat for the fat you do include in your eating plan.
  - —Keep saturated fat to less than 7 percent of calories. Any trans fats you eat are included in this scant amount.
  - —Instead of choosing foods high in saturated fats, substitute more foods with higher amounts of
    - monounsaturated fats
    - Omega-3 fats

Before I put all these factors into perspective and convert them into the food that goes on your plate, let's slide through a few fat facts.

All About Fat, a Most Confusing Topic

Our relationship with dietary fat is confusing. In the fervor to reduce dietary fat, Americans are forgetting a crucial fact: It is the dose that makes the poison. Consider this analogy: Aspirin can lower a fever and relieve pain at the right dose, but it is harmful at higher doses. The same is true of many nutrients and chemicals. Too much salt and even too much water can be fatal. But like fat, they are crucial to the human body. Let's take a look at the crucial roles fat plays in our body.

Without fat the body's billions of cells could not form properly because fat is an essential ingredient for cells. They could not regulate the entry and exit of nutrients, hormones, and other life-essential chemicals because fat-containing substances stand guard at the entry and exit of many cells. Vital internal organs might suffer serious injury in the absence of fat because fat cushions them. Hormones couldn't form or function without fat, and the body could not harness, transport, and use certain essential vitamins.

So why the confusion over dietary fat? You are not alone if you are asking: If I need this fat in every cell in my body, then why is fat in my food such a problem? While we definitely need some fat in our food to maintain healthy fat cells and to harvest the fat-soluble nutrients every cell needs to function, we have to be very careful with fat. Why? Because fat is the most calorically dense food substance we eat, supplying 9 calories per gram. That is two and one-quarter times the calories we get from an equal amount of carbohydrates and protein (which is why a little piece of fat-rich chocolate cheesecake can do so much damage). It is easy to run in to types of fat that increase the chances of developing artery-clogging heart disease, especially in America with so many convenience foods—and also so many fruits and vegetables missing in action.

The bottom line about fat: A little goes a long way.

The chemistry of fat. Chemically speaking, fat is just one substance in a larger category of substances called lipids. Oily or greasy to the touch and insoluble in water, lipids include dietary fats such as cooking oil, butter, lard, and the fat in many meats, dairy products, and other foods.

Is Cholesterol a Fat?

Cholesterol is not exactly a fat but falls under the lipid umbrella, that larger category of substances in which dietary fats exist. Cholesterol is one example of a sterol, which is not dietary fat at all but a fatlike, waxy substance present in all animal cells and made in the liver.

This is a very important point: Cholesterol is found only in foods of animal origin, simply because it is made by the liver. Even totally fat foods from plant sources, such as olive oil, canola oil, and walnuts, cannot have cholesterol.

Cholesterol does not supply calories because it is not composed of the same energy-supplying compounds that fats and oils are. Surprisingly, the majority of the cholesterol in our bodies is formed in the body itself, by the liver. Other substances included under the lipid umbrella, besides dietary fats and cholesterol, are hormones and waxes.

How nature makes fats.   Fat is formed from the same ingredients found in nature as are protein and carbohydrates: carbon, hydrogen, and oxygen. The difference is in the proportions and how the basic ingredients are connected. Fats contain much less oxygen than do carbohydrates and proteins (and fats do not contain any nitrogen, as proteins do). Simply put, the air is squeezed out of fat, which makes it a more compact source of energy. Although this is a simplification, it is why fats pack in so many more calories than carbohydrates and protein in an equal amount of weight.

Saturated fats and trans fats versus unsaturated ones.   Dietary fats consist mainly of building blocks called triglycerides. In turn, triglycerides are made up of one glycerol molecule connected to three fatty acids. The most important structural feature of a triglyceride is the fatty acid portion. This is the segment that distinguishes one type of triglyceride, or dietary fat, from the other, both in terms of flavor and the fat's effect in the body. Some fatty acids are saturated, some are monounsaturated, and others are polyunsaturated.

You hear so much about saturated versus unsaturated fats, and how important they are to your health. Fats are made up of carbon atoms, hydrogen atoms, and oxygen atoms. Saturation simply has to do with how much hydrogen a fat contains. Mother Nature did this fancy footwork with fats, allowing them to have different amounts of hydrogen atoms, and this is what defines their levels of saturation.

- Saturated fatty acids are saturated with hydrogen, or contain the maximum amount of hydrogen atoms possible.

- Fats missing one pair of hydrogen atoms are monounsaturated.

- Fats missing more than one pair of hydrogen atoms are polyunsaturated.

- And then there are trans fats (see sidebar), an invention of modern technology.

Although these fats differ by just a couple of hydrogen atoms, they do not behave the same in the body.

All foods have fats with all types of saturation. Any food that contains fat has all three types of fatty acids. Generally, though, one type of fatty acid predominates. So why are some foods called monounsaturated fats and some saturated fats?

This confusion stems from the fact that dietary fats are generally called by the name of the predominating fat. Olive oil, for example, is called a monounsaturated fat because 75 percent of its fatty acids are monounsaturated. However, it also contains some polyunsaturated and a little saturated fat. Even butter, which contains 62 percent saturated fat, has 30 percent monounsaturated fat.

Fats that are predominantly poly- and monounsaturated fatty acids are liquid at room temperature. Saturated fats are solid. Picture a bottle of liquid olive oil and a stick of butter at room temperature or the white waxy layer of saturated fat on a platter of cooling roast beef. These fats paint the same picture inside your arteries.

As a rule, fats of plant origin, such as vegetable oils, are almost entirely poly- and monounsaturated (the only two exceptions are coconut and palm oils, which are predominantly saturated fat). Animal fats—those in dairy foods, beef, pork, and chicken—are predominantly saturated. Marine fats, or fats from fish, are in a different category because they have some unique benefits to human health, especially to the health of diabetics. I will explain the special fat from fish in more detail later, but for now you should think of foods and the fat they supply in four groups:

1. Fats from plant sources
2. Fats from fish
3. Fats from animal sources
4. Trans fats

I am going to make a clear demarcation that is highly significant when it comes to choosing a better fat. Fats from plant sources and fats from fish sources are the best types for you. Fats from animal sources and trans fats are the worst. You will soon see that there is an absolutely clear connection to why I recommended that you eat your protein foods the way I did.

The Villainous Trans Fats

Trans fatty acids are created during hydrogenation, the process by which liquid vegetable oils are converted to solid or semi-solid shortening and margarine. Picture a bottle of canola oil and then canola oil margarine. Trans fats give products such as boxed cookies, crackers, cakes, and other convenience foods a longer shelf life.

Although they are created from heart-friendlier vegetable oils, trans fatty acids undergo more than a physical transformation: The way they affect the body also changes dramatically. Once "hydrogenated" or "partially hydrogenated," these fats act more like sinister saturated fats. A recent review in the journal *Nutrition Reviews* provided an excellent explanation of foods containing trans fats. World-renowned fat researcher Martijn B. Katan of the Wageningen Centre for Food Sciences and the Division of Human Nutrition and Epidemiology at Wageningen University in the Netherlands writes: "Perceptions of the health effects of trans-fatty acids, particularly in the form of margarine, have undergone several changes during the past 10 years. What was once heralded as the healthy alternative to butter now assumes the role of co-conspirator."

Indeed, there is no doubt that trans fatty acids increase total and LDL cholesterol levels. Trans fats also decrease levels of HDL cholesterol, the "good" cholesterol fraction that protects against heart disease.

One of the most forceful messages about the adverse effects of trans fatty acids came in 1994 when Harvard researchers Walter Willett and Alberto Ascherio conservatively estimated that thirty thousand deaths per year in the United States might be due to trans fats.

While it gets the most attention, margarine is hardly the most significant source of trans fats. Rather, it is the shortening used to make fast foods and convenience foods. In 1997 the per capita consumption of fat in the United States from margarines was 9.9 pounds a year, or about 12 grams per day. In contrast, we consumed on average 20.9 pounds of hydrogenated vegetable shortening, or about 26 grams per day. Here is a quick look at some trans fat facts: The shortenings used by many fast food establishments to make French fries, doughnuts, and other fried foods contain 11 to 34 percent trans fatty acids. Translating this to what you eat, a medium-size helping of French fries contains 5 to 6 grams of trans fatty acids.

The negative health consequences of consuming trans fatty acids is so strong that the U.S. Food and Drug Administration has proposed new rules for labeling foods with their trans fatty acid content. The FDA proposed that the Nutrition Facts Panel should include a footnote specifying the content of trans fat in that food. (If a food contains less than 0.5 gram of trans fat, however, there won't be a footnote, because analytical methods cannot reliably measure lower levels.)

In the meantime, you can reduce your intake of trans fatty acids by doing the following:

- Use liquid oils instead of solid shortenings and margarines.
- If you must use margarine, choose one that is trans fat free. You can tell this because the label will generally boast that it is. To be sure, though, read the ingredient list. If you see an ingredient beginning with "partially hydrogenated" or "hydrogenated," you'll know it contains trans fats. *Just because a product says "no saturated fat" or "no cholesterol" does not mean it is trans fat free, so read carefully.*
- Choose crackers, cookies, and other convenience products similarly, looking for the same terminology.
- Reduce or eliminate your consumption of fast foods, especially those that are fried.

These choices impact your fat intake, both the total amount and the type of fat. This is meant to make it easier to remember how to eat. In the protein chapter it was recommended that you choose plant sources of protein as much as possible at lunch time. For dinner it was suggested that in a given week you should have at least two fish meals, at least two vegetable sources of protein, and then either two poultry meals and one red meat meal or two red meat meals and one poultry meal—or more fish or vegetable sources of protein.

You should now appreciate why I made those recommendations in the last chapter. Let's take a look at one more important question before I move on to a more detailed discussion of saturated and trans fats versus unsaturated fats and their significance to your health.

Is there really such a thing as essential fats?   Absolutely. As you may recall from Chapter Five, there are nine essential amino acids that must be obtained through the diet. The body can make almost all fatty acids it needs from the scraps of carbon, hydrogen, and oxygen atoms left over from any excess fat, protein, or carbohydrate foods we eat. But three fatty acids— linoleic, arachidonic, and linolenic—cannot be made in the body and are therefore called *essential fatty acids.*

How much fat do we need each day to construct these essential fatty acids? Much less than most people consume. Just 20 grams of dietary fat— as polyunsaturated fats that have those three fatty acids—will meet the body's daily requirement. However, a diet this low in fat is not palatable for most people. In addition, an eating plan this low in fat would probably make it difficult to control blood sugars.

The real key when adding the needed extra fat is to choose it carefully, minimizing the saturated fat as much as possible and—for the sake of your diabetes—maximizing the choices that offer monounsaturated fats and the special category of polyunsaturated fats known as omega-3 fatty acids.

Avoid the Low-Fat Trap

Low-fat foods can be a wonderful addition to your eating plan—but only when used to replace their full-fat counterpart. Many people overuse these products, most of which are still high in calories (simple carbohydrate calories) and low in nutrients. Examples are eating a whole bag of low-fat cookies or chips, or a huge bowl of nonfat frozen yogurt. Not only do you end up with too many calories and too many carbohydrates, but you also come up terribly short on nutrients.

More on Saturated, Monounsaturated, and Polyunsaturated Fats

Why is saturated fat such an enemy to the heart and to a person with diabetes? Saturated fat is the heart's greatest food enemy. It is the most significant dietary culprit in raising blood cholesterol levels, especially the LDL cholesterol, the cholesterol fraction that builds up on arterial walls and narrows them. For every 1 percent increase in dietary saturated fat intake, serum cholesterol increases 2.4 mg/dl (milligrams per deciliter). Overall, saturated fats contribute about 11 to 12 percent of calories to the American diet. Because of their potent hypercholesterolemic nature (i.e., their ability to raise blood cholesterol levels), the American Heart Association (AHA) recommends limiting them to 8 to 10 percent of total calories, and to less than 7 percent in those who have high cholesterol levels or atherosclerotic heart disease. Because people with Type 2 diabetes have such a high risk of heart disease, they should limit saturated fat to less than 7 percent of calories.

One of the ways saturated fat is thought to raise LDL cholesterol levels is by impairing the liver's cholesterol removal machinery. In the best of all metabolic conditions, LDL receptors are like large grappling hooks on the ends of liver cells, ready to snag LDL cholesterol as it flows by. The LDL particles are then packaged for removal from the body via the intestinal tract.

Saturated fat, however, prevents the "grappling hooks" from working properly. In a simplistic sense, saturated fat gums up the works by both reducing the number of LDL receptors and impairing their efficiency. This is one reason that saturated fat is such a culprit in keeping LDL cholesterol too high.

Are both kinds of unsaturated fat—polyunsaturated and mono-unsaturated—okay? Substituted for saturated fat, polyunsaturated and monounsaturated fats are far superior for the heart. When you reduce your total fat intake and substitute unsaturated fats, you have a better chance of improving your lipid profile. While the prevailing opinion varies about what is better for the general population (that is, people without diabetes), health professionals strongly recommend that *as a diabetic you should strive to get the majority of your fat as monounsaturated fats.*

Research consistently reveals that people with diabetes who eat high-mono fat diets have improved lipoprotein profiles as well as better glycemic control. Research also shows that mono fats reduce fasting plasma triglycerides and VLDL cholesterol concentrations by 19 and 22 percent respectively. One more good thing that monos do is cause a modest increase in HDL cholesterol without adversely affecting LDL cholesterol.

A special note: Some people with very high levels of triglycerides in their blood may need special dietary adjustments. Sometimes there is a need to reduce the percentage of calories from carbohydrates, so they must raise the percentage of calories from fats. In such cases fats high in mono fats are the recommended way to go. This should only be done with a doctor's advice and with the help of a registered dietitian.

Omega-3 Fats: A Good Type of Polyunsaturated Fat

You can't help but noticing that I am keen on getting you to eat more fish, especially fish rich in omega-3 fats. Before I explain why these fats may help you, let me explain a little history about omega-3 fats as well as what they are.

The Greenland Eskimos first revealed to the world that eating fish might decrease heart disease risk. International research is now incredibly consistent in uncovering the same association: Death from heart disease is more unusual among people who eat at least some fish than among those who do not. For diabetics this might be especially important.

Surprisingly, it is the fat in fish that confers most of the benefit. Fish contain a special type of polyunsaturated fatty acids called omega-3. This special type of "body fat" helps fish adapt to the cold water in which they live. You may have even read about two of these omega-3s that are especially abundant in fish: eicosapentaenoic acid and docosahexaenoic acid.

By slowing the production of prostaglandins, leukotrienes, and thromboxanes, omega-3s stop the body's immune system from working overtime. While the body needs some of these chemicals to function normally, concentrations that are too high can lead to trouble. Just the right amount helps blood vessels contract and relax appropriately to control blood pressure, but too much makes blood vessels contract too forcefully, driving up blood pressure. An overload also encourages platelets to clump or aggregate overzealously, a risk factor for coronary artery disease (CAD) and heart attack. Omega-3s also raise HDL cholesterol. In fact, eating fish may keep HDL cholesterol from dropping, as it is known to do on a low-fat diet.

In addition to its favorable effects on platelets and HDL cholesterol, the oil in fish may keep the heart beating in a healthy rhythm. Although you are rarely aware of it, your heart beats an average of 72 times a minute, or over 100,000 times every day. Either out of fear or excitement, no doubt you have felt your heart "skip a beat" or race momentarily, but for the most part your heart beats evenly, in a steady rhythm, thanks to its sophisticated electrical system.

Sometimes, though, the electrical system goes awry, causing the heart to beat unevenly or out of rhythm. This is called an arrhythmia. While some arrhythmias are perfectly harmless, others are dangerous and can cause the heart to stop beating altogether (cardiac arrest). There is increasing evidence that omega-3 fatty acids may guard against dangerous arrhythmias, somehow fortifying the heart muscle against unstable beats. In a recent study, people who ate enough fish to get 5.5 grams of omega-3 fatty acids in a month—just one 3-ounce serving of salmon weekly—had only half the risk of cardiac arrest as people who ate no omega-3s.

Fish may also offer some protection for people who have already suffered one heart attack. There is now very good evidence that including at least two fish meals per week (each about 3 ounces) may reduce the chances of suffering a second, fatal heart attack. While all studies do not agree, it is also possible that fish can keep arteries from closing after angioplasty, a non-surgical procedure that opens blocked vessels in the heart.

Why you should focus on omega-3 fats. There is accumulating evidence that diets with omega-3 fatty acids are beneficial for many of the metabolic derangements associated with Type 2 diabetes, the so-called syndrome X or Reaven syndrome. Omega-3s may counteract the hypertriglyceridemia (high blood triglyceride levels), hypertension, and weight gain associated with this syndrome. It is well known that omega-3 fatty acids lower triglycerides by decreasing hepatic VLDL synthesis.

So now you know why it is strongly suggested that you include at least two fish meals per week, and in this book you will find lots of recipes to help you!

What about fish oil capsules? This is the question everyone asks: If eating fish is so good for the heart, should I take fish oil capsules? Unless a physician prescribes fish oil capsules for very specific metabolic issues, stick to the real thing—fish, that is. Fish oil capsules are a concentrated source of fat calories, and it is easy to overdo them, which simply drives up fat intake. While some fish fat is good, too much can cause an elevation in LDL cholesterol and also lead to weight gain. Also, taking fish oil capsules and then eating a hamburger has no benefit. You simply cannot erase the negative effects of eating too much red meat and saturated fat with a pill. In fact, when all is said and done, you will end up with quite an excessive number of fat grams.

Putting It All Together

Here is what you learned about fat:

- Reduce your total consumption of fat, aiming for no more than 30 percent of calories as fat.

- Reduce your intake of saturated and trans fats, aiming for no more than a total of 7 percent of calories from both, 5 percent if you have had a heart attack or have known atherosclerosis. Do this in the following ways:

—Use nonfat dairy products.

—Eat no more than two red meat meals per week; always trim away visible fat and use lower fat cooking methods (see sidebar).

—Reduce or eliminate convenience snacks and fast foods.

- Substitute better fats for the fats you do eat. These better fats are those highest in monounsaturated fats and high in omega-3 fats. Practically speaking, this means to:

—choose canola oil and olive oil for cooking. (You will learn more about this in Chapter Eleven.) See the chart below for more detailed information.

—enjoy appropriate portions of nuts that are high in mono fats, such as pecans, peanuts, and almonds.

- Avoid the low-fat trap (see sidebar, p. 101).

Lower Fat Cooking Methods

Stir sizzle: This is the lower fat way to stir-fry. You have two options: Avoid the use of oil altogether by coating a nonstick pan with vegetable oil spray. Add vegetable, chicken, or beef broth as needed for the moisture needed to stir-fry. Alternatively, start with a teaspoon or two of canola or olive oil, and then add broth as needed for moisture.

Baking: Convert cookie, cake, and quick bread recipes that call for oil, butter, or shortening into lower fat versions. In most cases you can substitute applesauce or pureed prunes for up to half the fat. Also use better fat for the fat you do use, such as olive or canola oil. If you do not like the taste of olive oil, use the light version because the flavor is lighter. However, be aware that it has the same number of calories as the other olive oil.

NUTS (PER 2 TABLESPOONS)

	Total Grams of Fat	Total Calories	% of Calories as Saturated Fat	% of Calories as Monounsaturated Fat	% of Calories as Polyunsaturated Fat	Grams of Omega-3 Fatty Acids	Bonus Nutrients
Almonds	9.1	103	6	47	18	0.06	Riboflavin (9%), Vitamin E (23%), Copper (10%), Magnesium (12%), Manganese (23%), Phosphorus (8%)
Brazil nuts	11.9	121	34	—	—	—	Iron (4%)
Cashews	10.0	120	15	—	—	—	Iron (5%)
Peanuts	9.1	107	10	35	23	0	Niacin (12%), Vitamin E (7%), Folate (7%), Magnesium (8%), Manganese (19%), Phosphorus (7%)
Pecans	9.6	96	8	52	27	—	Thiamin (7%), Copper (8%)
Pistachios	7.3	91	8	36	20	0.04	Thiamin (9%), B_6 (14%), Copper (11%), Manganese (10%), Phosphorus (8%)
Walnuts	8.2	82	8	11	60	1.14	

OILS (PER 1 TABLESPOON)

	Total Grams of Fat	Total Calories	% of Calories as Saturated Fat	% of Calories as Monounsaturated Fat	% of Calories as Polyunsaturated Fat	Grams of Omega-3 Fatty Acids	Bonus Nutrients
Almond	13.6	120	8	70	17	0	Vitamin E (27%)
Canola	13.6	120	7	59	30	1.27	Vitamin E (14%)
Coconut	13.6	117	87	6	2	0	
Corn	13.6	120	13	24	59	0.1	Vitamin E (14%)
Hazelnut	13.6	120	7	78	10	0	Vitamin E (32%)
Olive	13.5	119	14	74	8	0.08	
Palm	13.6	120	49	37	9	0.03	Vitamin E (15%)
Peanut	13.5	119	17	46	32	0	Vitamin E (9%)
Walnut	13.6	120	9	23	63	1.42	

OTHER FATS (PER 1 TABLESPOON)

	Total Grams of Fat	Total Calories	% of Calories as Saturated Fat	% of Calories as Monounsaturated Fat	% of Calories as Polyunsaturated Fat	Grams of Omega-3 Fatty Acids	Bonus Nutrients
Butter	11.5	102	62	29	4	0.17	Vitamin A (11%)
Canola margarine	11	100	14	50	27	—	Vitamin A (10%)
Light margarine	4.0	45	20	20	41	—	
Light mayonnaise	4.9	50	14	—	—	—	
Margarine	11.3	101	19	45	31	0.04	Vitamin A (11%), Vitamin E (9%)
Mayonnaise	4.9	57	11	20	41	0.29	

Chapter Seven

Why You Can't Live Without Exercise

There is absolutely no getting around this very clear fact: If you have diabetes or if you are at risk for diabetes, you must exercise. How much you move your body is at least as important as how you eat to control—and, it is hoped, minimize—your diabetes. In fact, in the days before there was insulin, regular exercise was the mainstay of therapy for people with Type 2 diabetes. Today, not only does exercise remain an important prescription in the treatment of diabetes, but also there is strong evidence that regular physical exercise protects against the development of Type 2 diabetes in high-risk populations.

You need to understand why exercise is so critical in your life and how to get started as soon as possible with an exercise routine you can maintain for a long, healthy life.

What Are the Benefits of Exercise for People with Diabetes?

It is hard to believe that a simple thirty-minute walk each day can save your life, but this could indeed be true for you if you have diabetes or are at risk for diabetes. A recent study published in the *Annals of Internal Medicine* reported on a group of men with Type 2 diabetes who were followed for twelve years in an attempt to ascertain the benefits of exercise. Some of the men exercised regularly, while others rarely exercised. After twelve years the physically inactive men were about twice as likely to die compared to the men who did exercise.

So what is it about exercise that so substantially improves the health of diabetics and even reduces the risk of death? Regular exercise:

- significantly improves blood sugars;
- reduces cardiovascular risk factors;
- helps reduce body weight and body fat;
- increases the sense of well-being.

Regular exercise significantly improves blood sugars. Exercising is nothing more than moving the muscles, which strengthens them. Officially this is called physical conditioning and is the phenomenon responsible for improving blood sugars and also decreasing insulin resistance.

When muscles are used regularly and more frequently, they are better able to use insulin. We call this increasing peripheral insulin sensitivity, where *peripheral* refers to the arms and legs. As you learned in earlier chapters, one of the problems in people with diabetes is insulin *insensitivity*. While the pancreas of a person with Type 2 diabetes can produce insulin, the cells are resistant to its effects. That is why people with Type 2 diabetes produce large amounts of insulin (with many ill effects, as you've learned).

Exercise has a wonderful chain of effects on blood sugars. It:

- increases peripheral insulin sensitivity;
- lowers insulin requirements;
- improves glucose tolerance;
- lowers blood sugars by increasing the uptake of glucose.

The effect of exercise lasts for several hours. Exercise produces increased glucose uptake in skeletal muscle, which means that blood sugars are improved for at least that long. Indeed, research has shown that a single exercise session can increase insulin sensitivity in liver and muscle tissue for up to sixteen hours.

While a single bout of exercise lowers blood sugars, regular exercise reverses one of the major abnormalities of Type 2 diabetes: It lowers fasting and postprandial insulin concentrations.

Timing exercise very specifically may have even greater benefits. Research has shown that postprandial (after a meal) exercise can result in a reduced post-meal blood glucose rise. Therefore, if you have Type 2 diabetes and experience hyperglycemia after eating, you may benefit from exercising one or two hours after meals. This will reduce blood glucose response to food consumed and certainly will minimize any risk of exercise-related hypoglycemia.

Regular exercise reduces cardiovascular risk factors. Regular exercise has two positive effects on cardiovascular risk factors:

1. It can lower blood pressure. Regular exercise, even without weight loss, can lower both the systolic and diastolic blood pressures (the top and bottom numbers) by five to ten points each.
2. It improves the lipid profile. Specifically, regular exercise raises HDLs, the good cholesterol fraction, and decreases three undesirable components: triglycerides, very low-density lipoproteins (VLDLs), and LDLs (what we commonly call the bad cholesterol fraction).

Regular exercise helps reduce body weight and body fat. Remember, it is critically important to achieve and maintain a leaner, healthier body in order to prevent the occurrence and decrease the severity of Type 2 diabetes.

Regular exercise increases the sense of well-being. Have you ever heard the expression "runner's high"? Well, that really should be "exerciser's high." Regular, sustained exercise causes the body to produce endorphins, natural body chemicals that are related to opiates. Not only do endorphins give you an increased sense of well-being by improving your mood, but they also help control pain, improve the immune system response, and improve the inflammatory response.

How Much Exercise Do You Need and How Often?

The bottom line, say diabetes experts, is that you should plan some form of physical activity five to seven days a week for twenty to forty-five minutes. This is optimal for improving blood sugar control and also managing weight.

Exercise must be something you enjoy, or you won't continue it. While you have probably thought of the conventional exercise options such as walking, cycling, swimming, and tennis, you should keep in mind that the following activities also constitute exercise: scrubbing floors, vacuuming, raking leaves, dancing, mowing the lawn, and washing windows. So if lack of time is one of your excuses, you can accomplish two things at once: Finish your chores and get in shape!

Can Exercise Adversely Affect Blood Sugars?

This is only a concern if you take insulin or pills to help control your blood sugars. If you do, you should discuss the appropriate timing of your exercise with a health professional.

Safety: A Key Concern Before and During Exercise

Safety is a key concern for every person who exercises, but it is of special concern for people with Type 2 diabetes for several reasons. First, as you've read repeatedly throughout this book, Type 2 diabetes raises the risk of heart disease. If you have been inactive for any period of time, you should have a thorough checkup by your physician before starting to exercise. Ask your physician if a stress test is appropriate for you.

You are also at increased risk of nonhealing sores, so it is important to avoid blisters and other foot injuries. Socks without holes or worn spots that can produce a blister and shoes that fit well and are not worn down in any one area are key components of exercise. Make sure there is a half-inch space between the front of your shoe and your big toe. If you have flat feet, you can remove the arch support inside the shoe. Your shoe should also have a wide heel, and the height should be about a half inch to prevent over-stretching your Achilles tendon.

To be on the safe side, inspect your feet before and after daily exercise.

Anyone who exercises—diabetic or not—can avoid complications by warming up before exercising and cooling down afterward, and carefully selecting an exercise type and intensity.

It is important to mention again that if you take insulin or pills to control your blood sugars, you must speak with your physician about timing your exercise appropriately so that your blood sugars do not fall too low.

Exercise Can Prevent Type 2 Diabetes

If you have Type 2 diabetes, then no doubt you have family members who are high risk. Or perhaps you are reading this book because you know you are at risk of developing Type 2 diabetes. This news is for you and your high-risk family members: Yes, exercise can prevent Type 2 diabetes, especially for those at high risk.

You see, exercise stops or at least improves the metabolic abnormalities that bring on frank diabetes. And research is abundant about the ability of exercise to prevent this dreadful disease.

In 1991 researchers studied former college students in the University of Pennsylvania Alumni Health Study. They found that those who exercised more were less likely to develop Type 2 diabetes in the fifteen years of follow-up.

Other studies have shown that the occurrence of Type 2 diabetes decreases by 6 percent for each increment of 500 calories burned per week in exercise. When men with the risk factors for diabetes (hypertension, obesity, and family history) were studied, it was found that physical activity had the greatest protective effect against getting the disease. Men in the highest activity group reduced their risk of diabetes by 24 percent compared to men in the lowest activity group.

If your doctor gives you the okay, get moving.
Every day is the best day to be active.

Chapter Eight

Twenty-eight Days of Menus at Your Calorie Level

You are ready to start a wonderful new way of eating every day. I've taken the guesswork out of all of this for you by providing twenty-eight days of meals at two calorie levels: 1,500 and 1,800. Consult your physician concerning the calorie level that is best for you. In general, though, I recommend 1,500 calories if you need to lose weight (which will help to make your diabetes disappear). If you are an appropriate weight, then 1,800 calories will probably work. Recipes for meals that appear in italics are in Chapter Twelve.

Remember: Portion control is key to all this! That means measuring spoons, measuring cups, and a scale are standard equipment in your kitchen, preferably in a place of honor on the counter so you are ready to use them every time you eat.

How to Use the Menus

These meal plans have many advantages:

- Every breakfast is exchangeable with every other breakfast. The same is true for lunches and dinners. This gives you endless possibilities for days' worth of meals.
- Each day has at least 25 grams of fiber and generally closer to 35 to 40. This gives you the best chance of eating away your diabetes. Be sure to add the veggies and legumes the meal plans call for.

- The saturated fat in these meals is extremely low, which gives you the best advantage of fighting heart disease. The secret is in following the portion sizes.

- Some of the recipes serve more than one. If you are cooking for one, you can either scale down the recipe or make the whole recipe and substitute it on another night in the same week. Or you can freeze the rest for later.

- In addition to the foods and amounts for each meal, you'll find calorie and nutrient totals. You'll also find exchanges or the number of servings from each food group.

Knowing these details, you can either follow the meal plans exactly as planned at your calorie level *or* mix and match the meals as you wish at your calorie level.

Day 1

Breakfast

Cinnamon-raisin-walnut oatmeal:
> 1 packet instant oatmeal
> ½ teaspoon cinnamon
> 2 tablespoons raisins

1 cup skim milk
2 tablespoons walnuts, chopped

Nutrition Totals 353 calories, 15.7 g protein, 49.3 g carbohydrates, 12.1 g fat

Exchanges 1.4 bread/starch, 0.3 lean meat, 1 fruit, 1 skim milk, 1.8 fat

Lunch

1 serving *Southwest Salad*
Seltzer water as desired

Nutrition Totals 504 calories, 25.3 g protein, 70.8 g carbohydrates, 16.1 g fat

Exchanges 3.2 bread/starch, 0.2 other carbs/sugar, 0.1 very lean protein, 3.1 vegetables, 1.8 fat

Afternoon Snack

1,500 Calories	*1,800 Calories*
1 serving *Zesty Cauliflower Salad*	1 slice *Kris's Highest Fiber (and Moistest) Bread* with 2 teaspoons peanut butter
98 calories, 4 g protein, 13.1 g carbohydrates, 3.9 g fat	459 calories, 23.2 g protein, 46 g carbohydrates, 21.2 g fat
0.2 bread/starch, 0.2 other carbs/sugar, 1.7 vegetables, 0.7 fat	1.8 bread/starch, 0.1 other carbs/sugar, 0.1 very lean protein, 1.2 lean meat, 1 skim milk, 3.4 fat

Dinner

1 serving *Pork and Pear Stew*
½ cup fat-free frozen yogurt with
> 1 cup fresh or frozen red raspberries

Nutrition Totals 497 calories, 33.7 g protein, 60.8 g carbohydrates, 12.2 g fat

Exchanges 1 other carbs/sugar, 3.4 lean meat, 2.3 fruit, 0.5 vegetables, 0.3 skim milk, 0.9 fat

Evening Snack

1,500 Calories
Herbal tea latté: Mix
    1 cup hot herbal tea
    with ½ cup skim milk

43 calories, 4.2 g protein,
5.9 g carbohydrates, 0.2 g fat

0.5 skim milk

1,800 Calories
1 serving *Berry Fresh Cheesecake*

222 calories, 15.6 g protein,
26.4 g carbohydrates, 5.6 g fat

0.4 bread/starch, 0.7 other carbs/sugar,
1.7 very lean protein, 0.4 lean meat,
0.2 fruit, 0.9 fat

Nutrition Totals for Day 1

	1,500 Calories	1,800 Calories
Calories	1,494	1,775
Protein (g)	83	98.3
Carbohydrates (g)	200	230.1
Fiber (g)	39	40.6
Fat (g)	44.5	55.4
Saturated Fat (g)	7.7	11.5
% Fat Calories	26	27
Cholesterol (mg)	85.9	99.7
Potassium (mg)	3,712	3,712
Sodium (mg)	1,799	1,792
Omega-3 Fatty Acids (g)	2.07	2.09
Exchanges	4.7 bread/starch	6.0 bread/starch
	1.4 other carbs/sugar	2.1 other carbs/sugar
	0 very lean protein	1.6 very lean protein
	3.4 lean meat	4.5 lean meat
	3.4 fruit	3.6 fruit
	5.2 vegetables	3.4 vegetables
	1.5 skim milk	1.1 skim milk
	5.1 fat	7.0 fat

Day 2

Breakfast

Raspberry smoothie: Blend
      1 cup fresh or frozen red raspberries
      8 ounces vanilla soy milk
      3 ounces firm lite silken tofu
1 slice *Kris's Highest Fiber (and Moistest) Bread*

Nutrition Totals 367 calories, 17.3 g protein, 57.3 g carbohydrates, 8.2 g fat

Exchanges 2.5 bread/starch, 0.1 other carbs/sugar, 0.8 very lean protein, 0.4 lean meat, 1 fruit, 1 fat

Lunch

1 serving *Black Bean and Artichoke Pita*
1 cup skim milk

Nutrition Totals 446 calories, 27 g protein, 67.5 g carbohydrates, 9.4 g fat

Exchanges 2.2 bread/starch, 0.3 other carbs/sugar, 1 very lean protein, 2.9 vegetables, 1 skim milk, 1.4 fat

Afternoon Snack

1,500 Calories	*1,800 Calories*
1 serving *Lemon Torte*	1 serving *Lemon Torte*
	1 cup skim milk
138 calories, 5.4 g protein, 26.6 g carbohydrates, 1.1 g fat	224 calories, 13.8 g protein, 38.5 g carbohydrates, 1.5 g fat
0.7 bread/starch, 0.8 other carbs/ sugar, 0.5 very lean protein	0.7 bread/starch, 0.8 other carbs/sugar, 0.5 very lean protein, 0.9 skim milk

Dinner

1 serving *Garlic-Sautéed Flounder and Vegetable Ribbons*
1 small baked potato with 1 teaspoon canola margarine
Spinach salad:
      3 cups fresh spinach
      4 mushrooms
      8 cherry tomatoes
      2 teaspoons olive oil
      1 tablespoon balsamic vinegar
      2 tablespoons fresh basil
¾ cup skim milk

Nutrition Totals 572 calories, 44.9 g protein, 56.1 g carbohydrates, 20 g fat

Exchanges 1.1 bread/starch, 3.9 very lean protein, 3.9 vegetables, 0.5 skim milk, 2.2 fat

Evening Snack

1,500 Calories	*1,800 Calories*
1 individual serving (4-ounce) "pop-top" can apricots in juice or water	1 serving *Trail Mix*
60 calories, 13 g carbohydrates	193 calories, 2.8 g protein, 24.8 g carbohydrates, 10.7 g fat
0.9 fruit	0.9 other carbs/sugar, 0.2 very lean protein, 0.7 fruit, 1.7 fat

Nutrition Totals for Day 2

	1,500 Calories	1,800 Calories
Calories	1,540	1,802
Protein (g)	89.3	105.8
Carbohydrates (g)	228.6	244.2
Fiber (g)	41.3	41.5
Fat (g)	32.6	49.8
Saturated Fat (g)	4.2	9.6
% Fat Calories	19	24
Cholesterol (mg)	93.7	101.4
Potassium (mg)	4,488	5,022
Sodium (mg)	2,200	2,053
Omega-3 Fatty Acids (g)	0.42	0.78
Exchanges	7.0 bread/starch	6.5 bread/starch
	1.9 other carbs/sugar	2.1 other carbs/sugar
	6.2 very lean protein	6.4 very lean protein
	0 lean meat	0 lean meat
	1.6 fruit	1.5 fruit
	6.6 vegetables	6.7 vegetables
	0.6 skim milk	2.3 skim milk
	4.4 fat	7.2 fat

Day 3

Breakfast

1 slice *Kris's Highest Fiber (and Moistest) Bread,* toasted, with
      2 teaspoons peanut butter
1½ cups skim milk

Nutrition Totals 327 calories, 20.4 g protein, 40.6 g carbohydrates, 10.2 g fat

Exchanges 1 bread/starch, 0.4 lean meat, 1.9 fruit, 1 skim milk, 1.7 fat

Lunch

1 serving *Goat Cheese and Brazil Nut Salad*

Nutrition Totals 542 calories, 33.9 g protein, 48.6 g carbohydrates, 26.5 g fat

Exchanges 0.4 bread/starch, 0.6 other carbs/sugar, 1.9 very lean protein, 1.9 lean meat, 4.4 vegetables, 4.1 fat

Afternoon Snack

1,500 Calories	*1,800 Calories*
1 fresh kiwifruit Seltzer water or sugar-free iced tea as desired	2 individual (1½-ounce) boxes raisins, mixed with 1 tablespoon dry-roasted almonds
50 calories, 1 g protein, 12 g carbohydrates, 0.5 g fat	313 calories, 3.9 g protein, 67.7 g carbohydrates, 4.7 g fat
0.8 fruit	0.3 lean meat, 4.3 fruit, 0.9 fat

Dinner

1 serving *Minted Orange Quinoa*
1 grilled or microwaved veggie burger*
1 cup fresh or frozen carrot coins, steamed, with
      4 large fresh or frozen broccoli spears
      2 teaspoons extra-virgin olive oil
      2 teaspoons lemon juice
1½ cups skim milk

Nutrition Totals 518 calories, 35.2 g protein, 68.6 g carbohydrates, 13.4 g fat

Exchanges 1 bread/starch, 0.6 lean meat, 0.2 fruit, 4.3 vegetables, 1.3 skim milk, 1.5 fat

---

BOCA Products have several wonderful varieties, from chicken-flavored to roasted onion.

Evening Snack

1,500 Calories	*1,800 Calories*
1 cup grapes	1 serving *Chocolate Silk Mousse*
114 calories, 1.1 g protein, 28.4 g carbohydrates, 0.9 g fat	98 calories, 5.5 g protein, 14.2 g carbohydrates, 1.2 g fat
1.9 fruit	0.3 bread/starch, 0.7 other carbs/sugar, 0.2 very lean protein, 0.4 lean meat

Nutrition Totals for Day 3

	1,500 Calories	1,800 Calories
Calories	1,551	1,798
Protein (g)	91.6	99
Carbohydrates (g)	198.2	239.7
Fiber (g)	27.8	31.3
Fat (g)	51.5	56.2
Saturated Fat (g)	15.8	16.1
% Fat Calories	29	27
Cholesterol (mg)	49.3	49.3
Potassium (mg)	4,299	4,642
Sodium (mg)	2,355	2,438
Omega-3 Fatty Acids (g)	0.40	0.34
Exchanges	2.5 bread/starch	2.8 bread/starch
	0.6 other carbs/sugar	1.3 other carbs/sugar
	1.8 very lean protein	2.1 very lean protein
	2.8 lean meat	3.4 lean meat
	2.9 fruit	4.3 fruit
	8.7 vegetables	8.5 vegetables
	2.8 skim milk	2.6 skim milk
	7.3 fat	8.0 fat

Day 4

Breakfast

2 egg whites, hard-boiled or scrambled
2 slices whole wheat bread with
      1 teaspoon canola margarine
1 cup fresh or frozen red raspberries
1 cup skim milk

Nutrition Totals 350 calories, 21.9 g protein, 52.6 g carbohydrates, 7.1 g fat

Exchanges 1.7 bread/starch, 1 very lean protein, 1 fruit, 1 skim milk, 0.8 fat

Morning Snack

1,500 Calories
Iced tea or coffee as desired

1,800 Calories
1 serving *Fudgey Brownies*
½ cup skim milk

211 calories, 7 g protein,
30.3 g carbohydrates, 7 g fat

0.3 bread/starch, 1 other carbs/sugar,
0.2 very lean protein, 0.4 skim milk, 1.2 fat

Lunch

2 servings *Caramelized Onion and Parmesan Bruschetta*
Easy salad:
      2 cups romaine lettuce
      1 carrot
      5 cherry tomatoes
      2 tablespoons low-fat salad dressing
1 fresh orange or 2 tangerines

Nutrition Totals 484 calories, 22 g protein, 68.6 g carbohydrates, 13.8 g fat

Exchanges 2 bread/starch, 0.3 other carbs/sugar, 0.6 very lean protein, 0.4 lean meat, 0.9 fruit, 3.6 vegetables, 0.5 fat

Afternoon Snack

1,500 Calories
1 large papaya

148 calories, 2.3 g protein,
37.3 g carbohydrates, 0.5 g fat

2.7 fruit

1,800 Calories
1 large papaya

148 calories, 2.3 g protein,
37.3 g carbohydrates, 0.5 g fat

2.7 fruit

Dinner

1 serving *Creamy Chicken and Rice*

Nutrition Totals 520 calories, 44.4 g protein, 51.1 g carbohydrates, 15.6 g fat

Exchanges 2.7 bread/starch, 5 very lean protein, 1.3 vegetables, 2.2 fat

Evening Snack

1,500 Calories
1 large sweet red bell pepper, sliced
3 leaves bok choy
2 tablespoons favorite salsa
(for dipping)

59 calories, 2.5 g protein,
13.5 g carbohydrates, 0.5 g fat

2.7 vegetables

1,800 Calories
2 tablespoons roasted pumpkin seeds

148 calories, 9.4 g protein,
3.8 g carbohydrates, 12 g fat

0.3 bread/starch, 1.2 lean meat, 1.3 fat

Nutrition Totals for Day 4

	1,500 Calories	1,800 Calories
Calories	1,561	1,861
Protein (g)	93.2	107
Carbohydrates (g)	223.1	243.7
Fiber (g)	40.4	38.8
Fat (g)	37.5	56
Saturated Fat (g)	7.5	12
% Fat Calories	21	26
Cholesterol (mg)	118.9	121.2
Potassium (mg)	4,219	4,269
Sodium (mg)	2,363	2,345
Omega-3 Fatty Acids (g)	0.69	0.72
Exchanges	6.4 bread/starch	7.0 bread/starch
	0 other carbs/sugar	1.1 other carbs/sugar
	6.5 very lean protein	6.8 very lean protein
	0.2 lean meat	1.3 lean meat
	4.3 fruit	4.2 fruit
	7.6 vegetables	4.8 vegetables
	0.6 skim milk	1.0 skim milk
	3.5 fat	6.1 fat

Day 5

Breakfast

8 ounces Breyer's Fat-Free Blueberries 'N Cream Yogurt with
    1 cup raspberries (fresh or frozen without added sugar)
    3 tablespoons dry-roasted almonds

Nutrition Totals 341 calories, 14.3 g protein, 41.1 g carbohydrates, 15.6 g fat

Exchanges 0.6 very lean protein, 1 fruit, 1.2 skim milk, 2.9 fat

Lunch

Veggie pita:
    1 whole wheat pita pocket
    ½ cup cucumber slices
    2 tomato slices
    ½ cup romaine lettuce
    2 tablespoons fat-free ranch salad dressing
Fruity cottage cheese:
    ½ cup 1% fat cottage cheese
    ½ cup canned pineapple
2 dried peach halves

Nutrition Totals 497 calories, 30 g protein, 64.1 g carbohydrates, 16.8 g fat

Exchanges 2.1 bread/starch, 0.7 other carbs/sugar, 2.8 very lean protein, 1.1 fruit, 0.8 vegetables, 2 fat

Afternoon Snack

1,500 Calories
4 ounces baby carrots with
¼ cup favorite salsa
Seltzer water as desired

61 calories, 1.8 g protein,
13.3 g carbohydrates, 0.8 g fat

2.5 vegetables

1,800 Calories
1 serving *Ginger-Poached Pears* with
4 ounces Breyer's Low-Fat Vanilla
Yogurt

168 calories, 5.3 g protein,
33.8 g carbohydrates, 1.8 g fat

1.4 other carbs/sugar, 0.8 fruit

Dinner

1 serving *Grilled Beef Fajitas*
Mandarin-artichoke salad:
    2 cups romaine lettuce
    4 ounces artichoke hearts (canned/jarred in water)
    ¼ cup grated carrots
    1 cup canned mandarin oranges

Dressing:

> 1 teaspoon olive oil
> 1 tablespoon balsamic vinegar
> 1 tablespoon lemon juice

Nutrition Totals 536 calories, 29.9 g protein, 72.3 g carbohydrates, 16.4 g fat

Exchanges 1.1 bread/starch, 0.3 other carbs/sugar, 2.5 lean meat, 0.9 fruit, 5.5 vegetables, 0.1 skim milk, 1.6 fat

Evening Snack

1,500 Calories
1 serving *Ginger-Poached Pears*

58 calories, 0.3 g protein, 14.9 g carbohydrates, 0.3 g fat

0.1 other carbs/sugar, 0.8 fruit

1,800 Calories
1 serving *Frozen Peach Shake*

195 calories, 13.8 g protein, 33.1 g carbohydrates, 1.3 g fat

2.2 other carbs/sugar, 0.3 fat

Nutrition Totals for Day 5

	1,500 Calories	**1,800 Calories**
Calories	1,494	1,799
Protein (g)	76.3	95
Carbohydrates (g)	205.7	257.8
Fiber (g)	39	39
Fat (g)	49.9	52.7
Saturated Fat (g)	8.6	10.4
% Fat Calories	28	25
Cholesterol (mg)	82	100.4
Potassium (mg)	3,519	4,303
Sodium (mg)	2,177	2,417
Omega-3 Fatty Acids (g)	0.45	0.45
Exchanges	2.9 bread/starch	2.9 bread/starch
	0.5 other carbs/sugar	4.0 other carbs/sugar
	3.0 very lean protein	3.0 very lean protein
	2.2 lean meat	2.2 lean meat
	3.8 fruit	3.8 fruit
	8.7 vegetables	8.7 vegetables
	1.2 skim milk	1.2 skim milk
	7.2 fat	7.8 fat

Day 6

Breakfast

1 serving *Sweet Pepper and Cheddar Cheese Scramble*
2 ounces whole wheat bagel
½ cup fresh or frozen strawberries

Nutrition Totals 386 calories, 25.1 g protein, 52.4 g carbohydrates, 10.3 g fat

Exchanges 2 bread/starch, 1.5 very lean protein, 2.2 vegetables, 0.9 fat

Lunch

1 serving *Turkey Tomato Wrap*
1 medium pear
1 Hershey's Chocolate Kiss

Nutrition Totals 471 calories, 33.2 g protein, 67.9 g carbohydrates, 11.8 g fat

Exchanges 0.9 bread/starch, 0.7 other carbs/sugar, 3.3 very lean protein, 1.7 fruit, 2.4 vegetables, 1.7 fat

Afternoon Snack

1,500 Calories	*1,800 Calories*
Herbal tea latte: Mix 　　1 cup hot herbal tea 　　½ cup skim milk	10 walnut halves 3 dried apple rings Green tea
43 calories, 4.2 g protein, 5.9 g carbohydrates, 0.2 g fat	179 calories, 3.3 g protein, 15.4 g carbohydrates, 13.3 g fat
0.5 skim milk	0.2 bread/starch, 0.4 lean meat, 0.8 fruit, 2.2 fat

Dinner

1 serving *White Bean and Tomato Pasta Sauce*
Spinach salad with
　　2 cups fresh spinach
　　5 cherry tomatoes
　　1 tablespoon chopped walnuts
Dressing:
　　1 tablespoon extra-virgin olive oil
　　1 teaspoon lemon juice

Nutrition Totals 523 calories, 15.6 g protein, 65.4 g carbohydrates, 23.9 g fat

Exchanges 2.5 bread/starch, 0.1 very lean protein, 2.6 vegetables, 4.1 fat

Evening Snack

1,500 Calories

1 chocolate-covered graham cracker
½ cup skim milk

111 calories, 5 g protein,
15.2 g carbohydrates, 3.5 g fat

0.6 other carbs/sugar, 0.5 skim milk,
0.5 fat

1,800 Calories

1 Chocolate Banana Balance Bar
1 cup skim milk

286 calories, 22.4 g protein,
33.9 g carbohydrates, 6.4 g fat

1.5 bread/starch, 1.4 very lean protein,
1 skim milk, 0.5 fat

Nutrition Totals for Day 6

	1,500 Calories	1,800 Calories
Calories	1,533	1,845
Protein (g)	83.1	99.5
Carbohydrates (g)	206.8	234.9
Fiber (g)	30.1	33.7
Fat (g)	49.6	65.7
Saturated Fat (g)	10.1	14
% Fat Calories	28	31
Cholesterol (mg)	83.4	88.4
Potassium (mg)	3,435	3,706
Sodium (mg)	2,071	2,237
Omega-3 Fatty Acids (g)	0.65	2.48
Exchanges	5.5 bread/starch	7.2 bread/starch
	0.6 other carbs/sugar	0 other carbs/sugar
	4.9 very lean protein	6.3 very lean protein
	0 lean meat	0 lean meat
	1.4 fruit	2.3 fruit
	7.2 vegetables	7.2 vegetables
	0.3 skim milk	0.3 skim milk
	7.3 fat	9.4 fat

Day 7

Breakfast

2 *Zucchini Fruited Muffins*
1 cup skim milk

Nutrition Totals 378 calories, 18 g protein, 65.7 g carbohydrates, 6.4 g fat

Exchanges 2.2 bread/starch, 0.3 other carbs/sugar, 0.2 very lean protein, 0.6 fruit, 1.1 skim milk, 0.9 fat

Lunch

1 serving *Ginger-Lentil-Barley Soup*
¼ cup soy nuts mixed with 1 tablespoon dried apricots

Nutrition Totals 472 calories, 29.6 g protein, 64 g carbohydrates, 13.4 g fat

Exchanges 3.2 bread/starch, 0.2 very lean protein, 1.8 lean meat, 0.2 fruit, 1.1 vegetables, 0.8 fat

Afternoon Snack

1,500 Calories	*1,800 Calories*

1 cup fresh or frozen red raspberries
½ cup skim milk
2 teaspoons Sugar Twin brown sugar
	1 carrot, peeled and sliced into sticks
	1 medium sweet green bell pepper, cored and cut into strips
	Vegetable dip: Mix
	    ¼ cup nonfat sour cream
	    Your choice of fresh herbs
	    Lemon juice to taste

106 calories, 5.3 g protein, 20.9 g carbohydrates, 0.9 g fat	107 calories, 4.1 g protein, 21.6 g carbohydrates, 0.2 g fat
0.1 other carbs/sugar, 1 fruit, 0.5 skim milk	2.9 vegetables, 0.4 skim milk

Dinner

1 Serving *Lemon Pepper Sizzled Tilapia*
½ cup brown rice, cooked
10-ounce package frozen asparagus spears or 20 fresh asparagus spears, steamed, drizzled with
    1 teaspoon olive oil
    1 teaspoon lemon juice
    Your choice of fresh herbs

Nutrition Totals 501 calories, 47.1 g protein, 38.5 g carbohydrates, 18.9 g fat

Exchanges 0.9 bread/starch, 5.2 very lean protein, 0.1 fruit, 2.3 vegetables, 2.8 fat

Evening Snack

1,500 Calories
1 serving *Vanilla Peach Mousse*

74 calories, 5.2 g protein,
13.5 g carbohydrates, 0.1 g fat

0.2 very lean protein, 0.5 fruit,
0.4 skim milk

1,800 Calories
1 serving *Ginger Snap Apple*

306 calories, 12.6 g protein,
42.7 g carbohydrates, 10.1 g fat

0.8 other carbs/sugar, 0.4 very lean
protein, 1.1 fruit, 0.7 skim milk, 1.8 fat

Nutrition Totals for Day 7

	1,500 Calories	1,800 Calories
Calories	1,531	1,764
Protein (g)	105.3	111.4
Carbohydrates (g)	202.5	232.5
Fiber (g)	39.5	37.5
Fat (g)	39.7	49
Saturated Fat (g)	6.8	7.8
% Fat Calories	22	24
Cholesterol (mg)	116.7	117.3
Potassium (mg)	4,152	4,814
Sodium (mg)	1,220	1,438
Omega-3 Fatty Acids (g)	2.28	2.65
Exchanges	6.1 bread/starch	6.0 bread/starch
	0 other carbs/sugar	0.4 other carbs/sugar
	5.9 very lean protein	6.1 very lean protein
	1.0 lean meat	0.9 lean meat
	2.4 fruit	2.0 fruit
	3.2 vegetables	6.4 vegetables
	1.2 skim milk	1.4 skim milk
	4.4 fat	6.4 fat

Day 8

Breakfast

1 *Blueberry Muffin*

Nutted yogurt:

   ½ cup favorite fat-free yogurt

   2 tablespoons soy nuts

Nutrition Totals 376 calories, 24.7 g protein, 49.8 g carbohydrates, 10.4 g fat

Exchanges 1.4 bread/starch, 0.1 other carbs/sugar, 0.1 very lean protein, 1.5 lean meat, 0.2 fruit, 1.2 skim milk, 0.7 fat

Lunch

Artichoke-chicken wrap:

   1 whole wheat tortilla

   4 ounces canned artichoke hearts

   3 ounces roasted chicken breast

   ¾ cup grated carrots

   1 tablespoon light mayonnaise

   1 teaspoon lemon juice

¼ cup dried cherries

Nutrition Totals 379 calories, 26.2 g protein, 59.6 g carbohydrates, 8 g fat

Exchanges 0.9 bread/starch, 0.1 other carbs/sugar, 2.3 very lean protein, 1.7 fruit, 3.0 vegetables, 1 fat

Afternoon Snack

1,500 Calories

Spinach-walnut stuffed pita:

   1 whole wheat pita pocket

   2 cups fresh chopped spinach

   2 tablespoons chopped walnuts

   ¼ teaspoon black pepper

   1 teaspoon balsamic vinegar

283 calories, 11.9 g protein, 40.3 g carbohydrates, 10.7 g fat

2.1 bread/starch, 0.1 other carbs/sugar, 0.5 very lean protein, 0.4 vegetables, 1.8 fat

1,800 Calories

Spinach-walnut stuffed pita:

   1 whole wheat pita pocket

   2 cups fresh chopped spinach

   2 tablespoons chopped walnuts

   ¼ teaspoon black pepper

   1 teaspoon balsamic vinegar

283 calories, 11.9 g protein, 40.3 g carbohydrates, 10.7 g fat

2.1 bread/starch, 0.1 other carbs/sugar, 0.5 very lean protein, 0.4 vegetables, 1.8 fat

Dinner

1 serving *Portobello Mushroom Caps with Caramelized Onions on a Bed of Quinoa*
1 Sugar-Free Jell-O Gelatin Snack
2 tablespoons Lite Cool Whip
1 cup strawberries

Nutrition Totals 501 calories, 16.2 g protein, 63.6 g carbohydrates, 16.8 g fat

Exchanges 2 bread/starch, 0.4 very lean protein, 0.8 fruit, 1.5 vegetables, 1.6 fat

Evening Snack

1,500 Calories
Herbal tea or café latté: Mix
    1 cup skim milk
    1 cup hot herbal tea or
    favorite flavored coffee

86 calories, 8.4 g protein,
11.9 g carbohydrates, 0.4 g fat

1 skim milk

1,800 Calories
1 serving *Fudgey Brownies*
1 cup skim milk

254 calories, 11.2 g protein,
36.2 g carbohydrates, 7.2 g fat

0.3 bread/starch, 1 other carbs/sugar,
0.2 very lean protein, 0.9 skim milk, 1.2 fat

Nutrition Totals for Day 8

	1,500 Calories	1,800 Calories
Calories	1,578	1,793
Protein (g)	95.5	100.2
Carbohydrates (g)	224.2	249.4
Fiber (g)	32.3	34.2
Fat (g)	41.8	53
Saturated Fat (g)	6.4	8.8
% Fat Calories	23	25
Cholesterol (mg)	77.8	77.9
Potassium (mg)	3,642	3,766
Sodium (mg)	2,424	2,509
Omega-3 Fatty Acids (g)	1.26	1.54
Exchanges	6.4 bread/starch	6.7 bread/starch
	0 other carbs/sugar	0.9 other carbs/sugar
	3.1 very lean protein	3.5 very lean protein
	1.0 lean meat	0.9 lean meat
	2.7 fruit	2.6 fruit
	4.9 vegetables	4.8 vegetables
	1.7 skim milk	1.6 skim milk
	4.2 fat	6.3 fat

Day 9

Breakfast

Nutty fruited yogurt:
> 8 ounces Breyer's Fat-Free Peaches 'N Cream Yogurt
> 2 tablespoons ground flaxseed
> 2 tablespoons soy nuts
> 2 dried apricots

Nutrition Totals 363 calories, 20.6 g protein, 48.5 g carbohydrates, 1.2 skim milk, 11.1 g fat

Exchanges 0.8 bread/starch, 1.5 lean meat, 0.8 fruit, 1.1 fat

Morning Snack

1,500 Calories
Tea or café latté: Mix
> 1 cup hot tea or coffee
> ½ cup skim milk

43 calories, 4.2 g protein,
5.9 g carbohydrates, 0.2 g fat

0.5 skim milk

1,800 Calories
Tea or café latté: Mix
> 1 cup hot tea or coffee
> 1 cup skim milk

86 calories, 8.4 g protein,
11.9 g carbohydrates, 0.4 g fat

1 skim milk

Lunch

Hummus-packed pita:
> 1 whole wheat pita pocket
> ½ cup hummus
> 4 ounces canned artichoke hearts
> 1 ounce mushrooms, sliced

1 cup skim milk

Nutrition Totals 478 calories, 25.9 g protein, 68.1 g carbohydrates, 14.1 g fat

Exchanges 3.4 bread/starch, 0.8 vegetables, 0.9 skim milk, 2.4 fat

Afternoon Snack

1,500 Calories
1 celery stalk, sliced, topped with
> 1 teaspoon peanut butter

38 calories, 1.6 g protein,
2.5 g carbohydrates, 2.8 g fat

0.1 lean meat, 0.3 vegetables, 0.5 fat

1,800 Calories
1 celery stalk, sliced, topped with
> 2 teaspoons peanut butter
> 1 mini (½-ounce) box raisins

80 calories, 2.1 g protein,
13.6 g carbohydrates, 2.8 g fat

0.1 lean meat, 0.7 fruit, 0.3 vegetables,
0.5 fat

Dinner

1 serving *Oven-Fried Chicken*
1 cup frozen peas and carrots with
    2 teaspoons canola margarine
1 cup fresh or frozen strawberries with
    2 tablespoons Lite Cool Whip

Nutrition Totals 523 calories, 44.2 g protein, 61.9 g carbohydrates, 16.6 g fat

Exchanges 0.8 bread/starch, 5 very lean protein, 0.8 fruit, 2.6 vegetables, 2.3 fat

Evening Snack

1,500 Calories
1 individual serving (8.25-ounce)
"pop-top" can light peaches

120 calories, 0 protein,
30 g carbohydrates, 0 fat

1.9 fruit

1,800 Calories
1 individual serving (8.25-ounce)
    "pop-top" can light peaches
2 tablespoons chopped walnuts

215 calories, 3.8 g protein,
31.9 g carbohydrates, 8.8 g fat

0.5 very lean protein, 1.9 fruit, 1.8 fat

Nutrition Totals for Day 9

	1,500 Calories	1,800 Calories
Calories	1,566	1,825
Protein (g)	96.5	105.8
Carbohydrates (g)	217	247.9
Fiber (g)	44.7	47.8
Fat (g)	44.7	56.5
Saturated Fat (g)	5.4	6.7
% Fat Calories	24	26
Cholesterol (mg)	103.8	106
Potassium (mg)	2,888	3,428
Sodium (mg)	2,396	2,484
Omega-3 Fatty Acids (g)	0.78	1.30
Exchanges	4.9 bread/starch	4.9 bread/starch
	0 other carbs/sugar	0 other carbs/sugar
	5.0 very lean protein	5.5 very lean protein
	1.1 lean meat	1.4 lean meat
	3.6 fruit	4.3 fruit
	3.7 vegetables	3.7 vegetables
	2.1 skim milk	2.6 skim milk
	6.3 fat	8.6 fat

Day 10

Breakfast

1 cup Raisin Bran cereal with
    1 cup skim milk
    2 tablespoons dry-roasted almonds

Nutrition Totals 376 calories, 16.7 g protein, 60.4 g carbohydrates, 11.3 g fat

Exchanges 2.7 other carbs/sugar, 0.4 very lean protein, 1 skim milk, 2 fat

Morning Snack

1,500 Calories	*1,800 Calories*
Omit	Tea or café latté: Mix
	1 cup hot tea or coffee
	1 cup skim milk
	86 calories, 8.4 g protein, 11.9 g carbohydrates, 0.4 g fat
	1 skim milk

Lunch

1 serving *Spinach and Barley Salad*
1 cup skim milk

Nutrition Totals 469 calories, 22.3 g protein, 66.6 g carbohydrates, 16 g fat

Exchanges 1.8 bread/starch, 0.1 other carbs/sugar, 4.6 vegetables, 1 skim milk, 2.6 fat

Afternoon Snack

1,500 Calories	*1,800 Calories*
1 fresh orange	1 medium orange
	1 kiwifruit
62 calories, 1.2 g protein, 15.4 g carbohydrates, 0.2 g fat	112 calories, 2.2 g protein, 27.4 g carbohydrates, 0.7 g fat
1 fruit	1.8 fruit

Dinner

1 serving *Lemon-and-Orange-Roasted Red Snapper*
1 cup green peas with
    1 teaspoon canola margarine

1 medium sweet potato, baked, with
    2 teaspoons Sugar Twin brown sugar
    1 tablespoon chopped walnuts
3 fresh apricots or 6 canned apricot halves

Nutrition Totals 521 calories, 29.6 g protein, 67.7 g carbohydrates, 16 g fat

Exchanges 3.2 bread/starch, 2.4 very lean protein, 1 fruit, 2.8 fat

Evening Snack

1,500 Calories	*1,800 Calories*
1 ounce toasted sesame breadsticks	1 ounce toasted sesame breadsticks with 1 tablespoon peanut butter
120 calories, 3.1 g protein, 17.9 g carbohydrates, 4 g fat	215 calories, 7.2 g protein, 21 g carbohydrates, 12.1 g fat
1.2 bread/starch, 0.5 fat	1.2 bread/starch, 0.4 lean meat, 2.1 fat

Nutrition Totals for Day 10

	1,500 Calories	**1,800 Calories**
Calories	1,548	1,779
Protein (g)	72.8	86.2
Carbohydrates (g)	228	254.9
Fiber (g)	44.4	47.3
Fat (g)	47.5	56.6
Saturated Fat (g)	6.4	8.3
% Fat Calories	26	27
Cholesterol (mg)	36.8	41.2
Potassium (mg)	4,822	5,575
Sodium (mg)	1,281	1,482
Omega-3 Fatty Acids (g)	0.9	0.92
Exchanges	6.2 bread/starch	6.2 bread/starch
	2.6 other carbs/sugar	2.6 other carbs/sugar
	2.8 very lean protein	2.8 very lean protein
	0 lean meat	0.1 lean meat
	2.0 fruit	2.8 fruit
	4.4 vegetables	4.4 vegetables
	1.7 skim milk	2.7 skim milk
	7.9 fat	9.5 fat

Day 11

Breakfast

1 serving *Cinnamon French Toast* with 1 tablespoon low-calorie pancake syrup
1 cup skim milk

Nutrition Totals 361 calories, 22.2 g protein, 45.6 g carbohydrates, 9.74 g fat

Exchanges 1.6 bread/starch, 0.5 other carbs/sugar, 1.1 very lean protein, 1 skim milk, 1.4 fat

Morning Snack

1,500 Calories	*1,800 Calories*
Omit	1 serving *Vanilla Peach Mousse*
	74 calories, 5.2 g protein, 13.5 g carbohydrates, 0.1 g fat
	0.2 very lean protein, 0.5 fruit, 0.4 skim milk

Lunch

1 serving *Chicken Caesar Salad*
1 cup grapes

Nutrition Totals 466 calories, 32.9 g protein, 68.7 g carbohydrates, 10 g fat

Exchanges 0.4 bread/starch, 0.1 other carbs/sugar, 2.3 very lean protein, 0.9 lean meat, 1.9 fruit, 4.2 vegetables, 0.9 fat

Afternoon Snack

1,500 Calories	*1,800 Calories*
1 medium banana	1 Chocolate Jell-O Fat-Free Pudding Snack (4 ounces) with 2 tablespoons Lite Cool Whip
109 calories, 1.2 g protein, 27.6 g carbohydrates, 0.6 g fat	181 calories, 3 g protein, 30.7 g carbohydrates, 6.2 g fat
1.9 fruit	1.9 other carbs/sugar, 1 fat

Dinner

1 serving *Stuffed Cabbage Casserole*
1 cup frozen carrots heated and served with 2 teaspoons canola margarine
1½ cups fresh or frozen red raspberries
½ cup skim milk

Nutrition Totals 513 calories, 37.9 g protein, 69.3 g carbohydrates, 12.9 g fat

Exchanges 0.4 bread/starch, 1 other carbs/sugar, 2.7 very lean protein, 1.2 fruit, 3.7 vegetables, 0.2 skim milk, 2.1 fat

Evening Snack

1,500 Calories
1 serving *Vanilla Peach Mousse*

74 calories, 5.2 g protein,
13.5 g carbohydrates, 0.1 g fat

0.2 very lean protein, 0.5 fruit,
0.4 skim milk

1,800 Calories
1 serving *Berry Fresh Cheesecake*

222 calories, 15.6 g protein,
26.4 g carbohydrates, 5.6 g fat

0.4 bread/starch, 0.7 other carbs/sugar,
1.7 very lean protein, 0.4 lean meat,
0.2 fruit, 0.9 fat

Nutrition Totals for Day 11

	1,500 Calories	**1,800 Calories**
Calories	1,523	1,817
Protein (g)	99.4	116.8
Carbohydrates (g)	224.8	254.2
Fiber (g)	49.7	49
Fat (g)	33.3	44.4
Saturated Fat (g)	7.5	13.9
% Fat Calories	19	21
Cholesterol (mg)	68.6	89.2
Potassium (mg)	5,369	5,424
Sodium (mg)	2,375	3,084
Omega-3 Fatty Acids (g)	1.86	1.93
Exchanges	2.3 bread/starch	2.7 bread/starch
	1.5 other carbs/sugar	4.1 other carbs/sugar
	6.3 very lean protein	8.0 very lean protein
	0.9 lean meat	0.9 lean meat
	5.5 fruit	3.9 fruit
	7.8 vegetables	7.6 vegetables
	1.6 skim milk	1.5 skim milk
	4.3 fat	6.1 fat

Day 12

Breakfast

1 serving *Cheesy Mushroom Omelet Wrap*
1 tangerine

Nutrition Totals 383 calories, 29.9 g protein, 53.4 g carbohydrates, 5.9 g fat

Exchanges 2.1 bread/starch, 2 very lean protein, 0.6 fruit, 1.1 vegetables

Morning Snack

1,500 Calories
1 carrot, sliced
Salsa as desired

35 calories, 1 g protein, 8 g
carbohydrates, 0 fat

1.4 vegetables

1,800 Calories
Omit

Lunch

1 serving *English Muffin Pizza*
1 cup fresh or frozen red raspberries topped with
     2 tablespoons slivered almonds
     ½ cup skim milk
     Brown Sugar Twin as desired

Nutrition Totals 464 calories, 25.7 g protein, 56.7 g carbohydrates, 16.9 g fat

Exchanges 1.7 bread/starch, 1.8 lean meat, 1 fruit, 1.2 vegetables, 0.5 skim milk, 2.3 fat

Afternoon Snack

1,500 Calories
2 bok choy stalks
Salsa as desired

4 calories, 0.4 g protein,
0.6 g carbohydrates, 0.1 g fat

0.1 vegetables

1,800 Calories
1 serving *Fudgey Brownies*

168 calories, 2.9 g protein,
24.3 g carbohydrates, 6.8 g fat

0.3 bread/starch, 1 other carbs/sugar,
0.2 very lean protein, 1.2 fat

Dinner

1 serving *Sesame Ginger Chicken Stir-fry*
½ cup brown rice, cooked
½ cup skim milk

139

Nutrition Totals 492 calories, 37.3 g protein, 65 g carbohydrates, 9.5 g fat

Exchanges 2.3 bread/starch, 0.1 other carbs/sugar, 3.2 very lean protein, 3.3 vegetables, 1.1 fat

Evening Snack

1,500 Calories
1 serving *Lemon Torte*

1,800 Calories
Peach smoothie: Blend
    8 ounces Breyer's Fat-Free Peaches 'N Cream Yogurt
    1 individual serving (8.25-ounce) "pop-top" can light peaches
    3 ounces extra-firm tofu
    Ice cubes

138 calories, 5.4 g protein, 26.6 g carbohydrates, 1.1 g fat

0.7 bread/starch, 0.8 other carbs/sugar, 0.5 very lean protein

272 calories, 14 g protein, 52.8 g carbohydrates, 0.6 g fat

0.9 very lean protein, 1.9 fruit, 1.2 skim milk

Nutrition Totals for Day 12

	1,500 Calories	**1,800 Calories**
Calories	1,517	1,815
Protein (g)	99.7	110.7
Carbohydrates (g)	210.3	260.2
Fiber (g)	43.5	43.5
Fat (g)	33.5	39.7
Saturated Fat (g)	7.2	9.3
% Fat Calories	19	19
Cholesterol (mg)	88.8	98.9
Potassium (mg)	3,194	3,103
Sodium (mg)	2,474	2,717
Omega-3 Fatty Acids (g)	0.43	0.42
Exchanges	6.8 bread/starch	6.4 bread/starch
	1.0 other carbs/sugar	1.2 other carbs/sugar
	5.7 very lean protein	6.3 very lean protein
	1.2 lean meat	1.2 lean meat
	1.1 fruit	2.9 fruit
	7.0 vegetables	7.0 vegetables
	0.4 skim milk	1.6 skim milk
	4.3 fat	4.7 fat

Day 13

Breakfast

2 *Carrot Date Muffins*
2 tablespoons soy nuts
1 cup skim milk

Nutrition Totals 356 calories, 20.9 g protein, 43.4 g carbohydrates, 12.4 g fat

Exchanges 1 bread/starch, 0.4 other carbs/sugar, 0.1 very lean protein, 1.2 lean meat, 0.5 fruit, 0.2 vegetables, 0.9 skim milk, 1.4 fat

Morning Snack

1,500 Calories	*1,800 Calories*
10 baby carrots	1 cup chocolate soy milk
38 calories, 0.8 g protein, 8.2 g carbohydrates, 0.5 g fat	120 calories, 4.6 g protein, 21.3 g carbohydrates, 2.3 g fat
1.6 vegetables	2.2 skim milk

Lunch

1 serving *Black Bean Soup with Cilantro*
8.25 ounces canned light apricots, sprinkled with 2 tablespoons sliced almonds

Nutrition Totals 476 calories, 16.9 g protein, 65.1 g carbohydrates, 16.8 g fat

Exchanges 0.6 bread/starch, 0.3 very lean protein, 0.8 lean meat, 1 fruit, 2.2 vegetables, 2.5 fat

Afternoon Snack

1,500 Calories	*1,800 Calories*
1 medium papaya	1 medium papaya
119 calories, 1.8 g protein, 29.8 g carbohydrates, 0.4 g fat	119 calories, 1.8 g protein, 29.8 g carbohydrates, 0.4 g fat
2.1 fruit	2.1 fruit

Dinner

1 serving *Southwest Tuna and Salsa*
½ cup instant brown rice
1 cup skim milk
4 Hershey's Chocolate Kisses

Nutrition Totals 570 calories, 48.2 g protein, 73.5 g carbohydrates, 10.3 g fat

Exchanges 2.1 bread/starch, 0.9 other carbs/sugar, 4.4 very lean protein, 0.1 fruit, 2.6 vegetables, 0.7 skim milk, 1 fat

Evening Snack

1,500 Calories
Omit

1,800 Calories
1 serving *Raspberry Cream Gelatin*

175 calories, 18.2 g protein, 23.3 g carbohydrates, 0.4 g fat

1 other carbs/sugar, 2.3 very lean protein, 0.5 fruit

Nutrition Totals for Day 13

	1,500 Calories	**1,800 Calories**
Calories	1,559	1,825
Protein (g)	88.8	111.1
Carbohydrates (g)	220	258.2
Fiber (g)	29.9	32.3
Fat (g)	40.5	42.9
Saturated Fat (g)	8.3	8.2
% Fat Calories	23	21
Cholesterol (mg)	81.4	87.5
Potassium (mg)	5,141	5,031
Sodium (mg)	1,266	1,823
Omega-3 Fatty Acids (g)	1.13	1.16
Exchanges	3.4 bread/starch	3.5 bread/starch
	1.1 other carbs/sugar	2.0 other carbs/sugar
	4.8 very lean protein	7.1 very lean protein
	1.7 lean meat	1.5 lean meat
	3.6 fruit	4.1 fruit
	6.7 vegetables	4.9 vegetables
	1.4 skim milk	3.5 skim milk
	4.9 fat	4.7 fat

Day 14

Breakfast

1 serving *Nutty Irish Oatmeal*

Nutrition Totals 327.7 calories, 13.6 g protein, 48.92 g carbohydrates, 10.6 g fat

Exchanges 3.1 bread/starch, 0.1 other carbs/sugar, 0.6 lean meat, 0.1 vegetables, 0.9 fat

Morning Snack

1,500 Calories
Omit

1,800 Calories
1 cup grapes
2 tablespoons dry-roasted peanuts

220 calories, 5.4 g protein,
32.4 g carbohydrates, 10 g fat

0.3 bread/starch, 0.5 lean meat, 1.9 fruit,
1.3 fat

Lunch

1 serving *Mandarin Bulgur Salad*
½ cup skim milk

Nutrition Totals 468 calories, 21 g protein, 72.8 g carbohydrates, 13 g fat

Exchanges 2.6 bread/starch, 0.4 very lean protein, 0.3 lean meat, 1.2 fruit, 1.5 vegetables, 0.5 skim milk, 1.6 fat

Afternoon Snack

1,500 Calories
1 cup grapes

114 calories, 1.1 g protein,
28.4 g carbohydrates, 0.9 g fat

1.9 fruit

1,800 Calories
1 cup chocolate soy milk

120 calories, 4.6 g protein,
21.3 g carbohydrates, 2.3 g fat

2.2 skim milk

Dinner

1 serving *Barbecue Meat Loaf*
1 medium baked potato with
     1 tablespoon fat-free sour cream
     Your choice fresh herbs
1 cup fresh or frozen green peas, steamed, with
     1 teaspoon chopped parsley
     2 teaspoons lemon juice

Nutrition Totals 521 calories, 37.9 g protein, 64.7 g carbohydrates, 12 g fat

Exchanges 3.6 bread/starch, 0.1 other carbs/sugar, 0.2 very lean protein, 3.3 lean meat, 0.4 vegetables, 0.3 fat

Evening Snack

1,500 Calories	*1,800 Calories*
1 cup chocolate soy milk	2 Fig Newtons
	Tea as desired
120 calories, 4.6 g protein, 21.3 g carbohydrates, 2.3 g fat	120 calories, 2 g protein, 20 g carbohydrates, 3 g fat
2.2 skim milk	1.4 other carbs/sugar, 0.6 fat

Nutrition Totals for Day 14

	1,500 Calories	1,800 Calories
Calories	1,560	1,787
Protein (g)	78.6	84.9
Carbohydrates (g)	237.8	261.7
Fiber (g)	34.9	38.4
Fat (g)	39.2	51.2
Saturated Fat (g)	7.6	9.8
% Fat Calories	22	25
Cholesterol (mg)	44.9	44.9
Potassium (mg)	3,299	3,499
Sodium (mg)	605	726
Omega-3 Fatty Acids (g)	2.42	2.42
Exchanges	9.3 bread/starch	9.5 bread/starch
	0.3 other carbs/sugar	1.7 other carbs/sugar
	0.1 very lean protein	0.1 very lean protein
	4.2 lean meat	4.7 lean meat
	2.5 fruit	2.5 fruit
	2.0 vegetables	2.0 vegetables
	2.2 skim milk	2.2 skim milk
	2.8 fat	4.7 fat

Day 15

Breakfast

1 serving *Banana-Walnut Oatmeal*

Nutrition Totals 339 calories, 13.8 g protein, 54.1 g carbohydrates, 9.2g fat

Exchanges 1.7 bread/starch, 0.2 very lean protein, 0.7 lean meat, 1.9 fruit, 0.9 fat

Morning Snack

1,500 Calories	*1,800 Calories*

Hot cocoa: Mix
    1 cup skim milk
    2 tablespoons unsweetened
    cocoa powder
    Artificial sweetener
	1 serving *Apricot Cream* with
	    2 tablespoons chopped walnuts

110 calories, 10.5 g protein, 17.7 g carbohydrates, 1.9 g fat	183 calories, 14.3 g protein, 13.4 g carbohydrates, 9.1 g fat
0.2 bread/starch, 1.0 skim milk, 0.1 fat	1.8 very lean protein, 0.6 fruit, 1.6 fat

Lunch

1 serving *Fresh Vegetable and Lentil Salad*
¼ cup dried peaches

Nutrition Totals 437 calories, 15.9 g protein, 66 g carbohydrates, 15.6 g fat

Exchanges 1.3 bread/starch, 0.2 very lean protein, 1.6 fruit, 4 vegetables, 2.8 fat

Afternoon Snack

1,500 Calories	*1,800 Calories*

1 large sweet red bell pepper,
  sliced into strips
2 tablespoons salsa
	1 large sweet red bell pepper,
	  sliced into strips
	2 tablespoons salsa

53 calories, 1.9 g protein, 12.6 g carbohydrates, 0.4 g fat	53 calories, 1.9 g protein, 12.6 g carbohydrates, 0.4 g fat
2.5 vegetables	2.5 vegetables

Dinner

1 serving *Rosemary-Horseradish–Potato-Encrusted Chilean Sea Bass*
1 cup blueberries, topped with
    3 tablespoons soy nuts

Nutrition Totals 549 calories, 42.4 g protein, 62.3 g carbohydrates, 16.3 g fat

Exchanges 2.6 bread/starch, 3.2 very lean protein, 1.9 lean meat, 1.1 fruit, 1.2 fat

Evening Snack

1,500 Calories
Omit

1,800 Calories
Hot cocoa: Mix
    1 cup skim milk
    2 tablespoons unsweetened
    cocoa powder
    Artificial sweetener
    2 Fig Newtons

230 calories, 12.5 g protein,
37.7 g carbohydrates, 4.9 g fat

0.2 bread/starch, 1.4 other carbs/sugar,
1 skim milk, 0.7 fat

Nutrition Totals for Day 15

	1,500 Calories	1,800 Calories
Calories	1,489	1,792
Protein (g)	84.5	100.8
Carbohydrates (g)	212.7	246.1
Fiber (g)	41.1	46.2
Fat (g)	43.3	55.4
Saturated Fat (g)	9.9	11.5
% Fat Calories	25	26
Cholesterol (mg)	68.9	75.1
Potassium (mg)	5,360	5,843
Sodium (mg)	740	1094
Omega-3 Fatty Acids (g)	1.96	2.48
Exchanges	5.8 bread/starch	5.6 bread/starch
	0 other carbs/sugar	1.0 other carbs/sugar
	3.6 very lean protein	5.4 very lean protein
	2.6 lean meat	2.5 lean meat
	4.6 fruit	5.1 fruit
	6.5 vegetables	6.3 vegetables
	0.7 skim milk	0.6 skim milk
	5.0 fat	7.2 fat

Day 16

Breakfast

Apricot smoothie: Blend
>1 individual can (8.25 ounces) apricots
>8 ounces plain low-fat yogurt
>6 ice cubes
6 walnut halves

Nutrition Totals 351 calories, 15.2 g protein, 50.6 g carbohydrates, 8.6 g fat

Exchanges 0.2 bread/starch, 0.8 very lean protein, 0.2 lean meat, 0.9 fruit, 1.2 skim milk, 1.3 fat

Morning Snack

1,500 Calories
Omit

1,800 Calories
Hot cocoa:
>1 cup skim milk, warmed
>1 packet sugar-free hot cocoa mix
>(Use milk instead of water for a more satisfying, richer snack.)

133 calories, 12.1 g protein, 20.4 g carbohydrates, 0.9 g fat

0.6 other carbs/sugar, 1 skim milk, 0.1 fat

Lunch

1 serving *Sun-Dried Tomato and Tuna Quiche*
½ cup grapes
1 *Blueberry Muffin*

Nutrition Totals 478 calories, 33.1 g protein, 67.4 g carbohydrates, 10.1 g fat

Exchanges 2 bread/starch, 2.7 very lean protein, 0.1 lean meat, 0.4 fruit, 3.1 vegetables, 0.3 skim milk, 1.3 fat

Afternoon Snack

1,500 Calories
1 kiwifruit

50 calories, 1 g protein, 12 g carbohydrates, 0.5 g fat

0.8 fruit

1,800 Calories
1 kiwifruit
3 tablespoons soy nuts

195 calories, 13.8 g protein, 22.6 g carbohydrates, 7.5 g fat

0.7 bread/starch, 1.5 lean meat, 0.8 fruit, 0.1 fat

147

Dinner

1 serving *Peanut Quinoa Pilaf,* on a bed of
    2 cups fresh spinach
1 veggie burger patty
2 fresh apricots or 4 halves canned in juice
1 cup skim milk

Nutrition Totals 516 calories, 37 g protein, 65.4 g carbohydrates, 13.4 g fat

Exchanges 2.3 bread/starch, 0.9 very lean protein, 0.5 lean meat, 0.8 fruit, 0.7 vegetables, 0.5 skim milk, 1.4 fat

Evening Snack

1,500 Calories	*1,800 Calories*
1 medium apple with	1 medium apple with
1 teaspoon peanut butter	2 teaspoons peanut butter
113 calories, 1.6 g protein, 22.1 g carbohydrates, 3.2 g fat	145 calories, 3 g protein, 23.1 g carbohydrates, 5.9 g fat
0.1 lean meat, 1.4 fruit, 0.5 fat	0.3 lean meat, 1.4 fruit, 1.1 fat

Nutrition Totals for Day 16

	1,500 Calories	1,800 Calories
Calories	1,507	1,817
Protein (g)	87.9	114.2
Carbohydrates (g)	217.4	249.4
Fiber (g)	29.9	33.2
Fat (g)	35.9	46.5
Saturated Fat (g)	5.5	7.6
% Fat Calories	21	22
Cholesterol (mg)	31.1	36.7
Potassium (mg)	4,126	5,413
Sodium (mg)	2,786	3,106
Omega-3 Fatty Acids (g)	1.5	1.98
Exchanges	4.5 bread/starch	5.2 bread/starch
	0 other carbs/sugar	0 other carbs/sugar
	3.8 very lean protein	3.8 very lean protein
	1.0 lean meat	2.6 lean meat
	4.3 fruit	4.3 fruit
	3.8 vegetables	3.8 vegetables
	2.0 skim milk	2.9 skim milk
	4.6 fat	5.4 fat

Day 17

Breakfast

1 whole wheat English muffin with
    1 tablespoon peanut butter
1 cup skim milk
1 cup fresh or frozen strawberries

Nutrition Totals 364 calories, 19.2 g protein, 53.3 g carbohydrates, 10.6 g fat

Exchanges 1.7 bread/starch, 0.4 lean meat, 0.8 fruit, 1 skim milk, 1.6 fat

Morning Snack

1,500 Calories
Omit

1,800 Calories
2 Snackwell's Sugar-Free Lemon Crème
    Cookies
1 cup skim milk

169 calories, 9.3 g protein,
26.7 g carbohydrates, 4 g fat

0.7 other carbs/sugar, 1 skim milk, 0.7 fat

Lunch

1 serving *Quinoa Salad*

Nutrition Totals 457 calories, 25.3 g protein, 65.3 g carbohydrates, 14.3 g fat

Exchanges 2.0 bread/starch, 1.4 very lean protein, 0.3 fruit, 6.3 vegetables, 1.8 fat

Afternoon Snack

1,500 Calories
1 large sweet yellow pepper,
sliced into strips

50 calories, 1.9 g protein,
11.8 g carbohydrates, 0.4 g fat

1.9 vegetables

1,800 Calories
1 large sweet yellow pepper,
    sliced into strips
1 carrot, sliced into sticks
¼ cup fat-free sour cream with your
    choice fresh herbs

125 calories, 4.9 g protein,
25.8 g carbohydrates, 0.4 g fat

3.3 vegetables, 0.4 skim milk

Dinner

1 serving *Tomato-Barley Chicken Stew*

Nutrition Totals 454 calories, 34.6 g protein, 62.2 g carbohydrates, 7.6 g fat

Exchanges 2.0 bread/starch, 3.2 very lean protein, 5.4 vegetables, 1 fat

Evening Snack

1,500 Calories	*1,800 Calories*
½ whole wheat pita pocket stuffed with	½ whole wheat pita pocket stuffed with
1 cup romaine lettuce	1 cup romaine lettuce
1 teaspoon olive oil	1 teaspoon olive oil
135 calories, 4 g protein, 18.9 g carbohydrates, 5.6 g fat	135 calories, 4 g protein, 18.9 g carbohydrates, 5.6 g fat
1.1 bread/starch, 0.3 vegetables, 0.9 fat	1.1 bread/starch, 0.3 vegetables, 0.9 fat

Nutrition Totals for Day 17

	1,500 Calories	1,800 Calories
Calories	1,461	1,788
Protein (g)	85	97.3
Carbohydrates (g)	211.4	252.1
Fiber (g)	41.5	43.8
Fat (g)	38.5	51.8
Saturated Fat (g)	6.2	8.5
% Fat Calories	23	25
Cholesterol (mg)	67.2	71.6
Potassium (mg)	4,900	5,585
Sodium (mg)	2,065	2,396
Omega-3 Fatty Acids (g)	1.22	1.29
Exchanges	6.7 bread/starch	6.7 bread/starch
	0 other carbs/sugar	0.7 other carbs/sugar
	4.6 very lean protein	4.6 very lean protein
	0.1 lean meat	0.1 lean meat
	0.9 fruit	0.9 fruit
	13.8 vegetables	15.2 vegetables
	0.7 skim milk	2.1 skim milk
	5.4 fat	8.0 fat

Day 18

Breakfast

2 *Oat Bran Apricot Muffins*
1 cup skim milk

Nutrition Totals 326 calories, 15.8 g protein, 47.5 g carbohydrates, 8.7 g fat

Exchanges 0.9 bread/starch, 0.4 other carbs/sugar, 0.4 very lean protein, 0.2 lean meat, 0.8 fruit, 1.1 skim milk, 1.3 fat

Morning Snack

1,500 Calories	*1,800 Calories*
Omit	1 fresh orange
	62 calories, 1.2 g protein, 15.4 g carbohydrates, 0.2 g fat
	1 fruit

Lunch

1 serving *Hummus Spinach Wrap*
1 cup skim milk

Nutrition Totals 345 calories, 20.6 g protein, 53.9 g carbohydrates, 9.1 g fat

Exchanges 1.7 bread/starch, 1.8 vegetables, 1 skim milk, 1.6 fat

Afternoon Snack

1,500 Calories	*1,800 Calories*
1 banana	1 banana, embedded with 8 walnut halves
109 calories, 1.2 g protein, 27.6 g carbohydrates, 0.6 g fat	215 calories, 3.7 g protein, 29.9 g carbohydrates, 11.1 g fat
1.9 fruit	0.1 bread/starch, 0.3 lean meat, 1.9 fruit, 1.7 fat

Dinner

1 serving *Ginger-Seared Sole on a Bed of Ginger-Steamed Lentils*
Romaine-basil-artichoke salad:
      3 cups romaine lettuce
      4 ounces canned artichoke hearts
      1 teaspoon extra-virgin olive oil
      1 tablespoon balsamic vinegar
      1 teaspoon ground basil

Nutrition Totals 539 calories, 49 g protein, 66.2 g carbohydrates, 10.7 g fat

Exchanges 2.6 bread/starch, 3.6 very lean protein, 0.3 fruit, 3.6 vegetables, 1.5 fat

Evening Snack

1,500 Calories
1 serving *Fudgey Brownies*

168 calories, 2.9 g protein,
24.3 g carbohydrates, 6.8 g fat

0.3 bread/starch, 1 other carbs/sugar,
0.2 very lean protein, 1.2 fat

1,800 Calories
1 serving *Fudgey Brownies*
1 cup skim milk

254 calories, 11.2 g protein,
36.2 g carbohydrates, 7.2 g fat

0.3 bread/starch, 1 other carbs/sugar,
0.2 very lean protein, 0.9 skim milk, 1.2 fat

Nutrition Totals for Day 18

	1,500 Calories	1,800 Calories
Calories	1,487	1,740
Protein (g)	89.4	101.5
Carbohydrates (g)	219.5	249
Fiber (g)	43.8	48
Fat (g)	35.8	47
Saturated Fat (g)	5.4	6.7
% Fat Calories	21	23
Cholesterol (mg)	69.6	74
Potassium (mg)	4,324	5,038
Sodium (mg)	1,849	1,975
Omega-3 Fatty Acids (g)	0.46	1.94
Exchanges	5.6 bread/starch	5.7 bread/starch
	1.3 other carbs/sugar	1.3 other carbs/sugar
	4.2 very lean protein	4.2 very lean protein
	0 lean meat	0.2 lean meat
	2.9 fruit	4.0 fruit
	5.2 vegetables	5.2 vegetables
	1.7 skim milk	2.7 skim milk
	5.7 fat	7.4 fat

Day 19

Breakfast

1 cup Fiber One cereal with
    1 cup skim milk
    2 tablespoons almonds

Nutrition Totals 312 calories, 17.6 g protein, 62.4 g carbohydrates, 11.9 g fat

Exchanges 1.6 bread/starch, 0.4 very lean protein, 1 skim milk, 2 fat

Morning Snack

1,500 Calories
Omit

1,800 Calories
1 kiwifruit
8 ounces Breyer's Light Key Lime Pie
    Nonfat Yogurt

170 calories, 8.5 g protein,
34 g carbohydrates, 0.6 g fat

0.8 fruit, 1.2 skim milk

Lunch

Chicken salad pita:
    1 whole wheat pita pocket
    2 ounces chicken breast, roasted
    6 ounces canned artichoke hearts
    2 tablespoons chopped onions
    2 teaspoons extra-virgin olive oil
    1 leaf romaine lettuce
½ cup grapes
½ cup skim milk

Nutrition Totals 467 calories, 30.6 g protein, 60.1 g carbohydrates, 13.3 g fat

Exchanges 2.1 bread/starch, 2.3 very lean protein, 0.5 fruit, 2.2 vegetables, 0.5 skim milk, 1.9 fat

Afternoon Snack

1,500 Calories
1 kiwifruit

50 calories, 1 g protein,
12 g carbohydrates, 0.5 g fat
0.8 fruit

1,800 Calories
1 Rye Crispbread Wafer with 2 tablespoons hummus

83 calories, 3 g protein,
12.2 g carbohydrates, 2.8 g fat
0.7 bread/starch, 0.5 fat

Dinner

1 serving *The Best Tacos*
1 ounce low-fat baked tortilla chips with 2 tablespoons salsa

Nutrition Totals 448 calories, 21.8 g protein, 63.8 g carbohydrates, 14.1 g fat

Exchanges 1.6 bread/starch, 1.7 other carbs/sugar, 1.1 lean meat, 2 vegetables, 0.3 skim milk, 1.3 fat

Evening Snack

1,500 Calories	*1,800 Calories*
1 serving *Berry Fresh Cheesecake*	1 serving *Berry Fresh Cheesecake*
	1 cup fresh or frozen strawberries
222 calories, 15.6 g protein, 26.4 g carbohydrates, 5.6 g fat	300 calories, 16.5 g protein, 46.5 g carbohydrates, 5.8 g fat
0.4 bread/starch, 0.7 other carbs/sugar, 1.7 very lean protein, 0.4 lean meat, 0.2 fruit, 0.9 fat	0.4 bread/starch, 0.7 other carbs/sugar, 1.7 very lean protein, 0.4 lean meat, 1.6 fruit, 0.9 fat

Nutrition Totals for Day 19

	1,500 Calories	1,800 Calories
Calories	1,495	1,780
Protein (g)	86.2	97.9
Carbohydrates (g)	22	279.1
Fiber (g)	52.7	60.7
Fat (g)	45.2	48.5
Saturated Fat (g)	9.4	9.7
% Fat Calories	25	22
Cholesterol (mg)	70.9	82
Potassium (mg)	2,877	3,614
Sodium (mg)	2,735	2,980
Omega-3 Fatty Acids (g)	0.92	0.98
Exchanges	5.8 bread/starch	6.5 bread/starch
	2.5 other carbs/sugar	2.5 other carbs/sugar
	4.2 very lean protein	4.2 very lean protein
	1.5 lean meat	1.5 lean meat
	1.3 fruit	2.6 fruit
	4.1 vegetables	4.1 vegetables
	1.6 skim milk	2.8 skim milk
	6.0 fat	6.6 fat

Day 20

Breakfast

1 serving *Cinnamon Rice and Raisins*
1 cup skim milk

Nutrition Totals 379 calories, 18.7 g protein, 54.9 g carbohydrates, 10.1 g fat

Exchanges 1.1 bread/starch, 0.5 lean meat, 1 fruit, 1.5 skim milk, 1.7 fat

Morning Snack

1,500 Calories
Omit

1,800 Calories
1 fresh orange

62 calories, 1.2 g protein,
15.4 g carbohydrates, 0.2 g fat

1 fruit

Lunch

Peanut butter and banana sandwich:
    2 slices oat bran bread
    2 tablespoons peanut butter
    1 banana
½ cup skim milk

Nutrition Totals 483 calories, 19.7 g protein, 63.6 g carbohydrates, 19.8 g fat

Exchanges 1.6 bread/starch, 0.8 lean meat, 1.9 fruit, 0.5 skim milk, 3.5 fat

Afternoon Snack

1,500 Calories
3 tablespoons soy nuts

145 calories, 12.8 g protein,
10.6 g carbohydrates, 7 g fat

0.7 bread/starch, 1.5 lean meat, 0.1 fat

1,800 Calories
8 ounces Breyer's Fat-Free Strawberry Yogurt

120 calories, 8 g protein,
22 g carbohydrates, 0 fat

1.2 skim milk

Dinner

1 serving *Classic Spaghetti*
Broccoli-spinach salad:
    2 cups spinach
    1 cup raw broccoli florets
    5 cherry tomatoes

Dressing:
      2 teaspoons olive oil
      2 teaspoons balsamic vinegar

Nutrition Totals 520 calories, 29 g protein, 70.4 g carbohydrates, 16.5 g fat

Exchanges 2.1 bread/starch, 0.7 very lean protein, 1.2 lean meat, 6.9 vegetables, 2.2 fat

Evening Snack

1,500 Calories
1 kiwifruit

50 calories, 1 g protein,
12 g carbohydrates, 0.5 g fat

0.8 fruit

1,800 Calories
1 kiwifruit
3 tablespoons soy nuts

191 calories, 13.5 g protein,
21.9 g carbohydrates, 7.3 g fat

0.7 bread/starch, 1.5 lean meat, 0.8 fruit,
0.1 fat

Nutrition Totals for Day 20

	1,500 Calories	1,800 Calories
Calories	1,573	1,755
Protein (g)	81	90.2
Carbohydrates (g)	210.8	248.2
Fiber (g)	28.8	32
Fat (g)	53.7	53.8
Saturated Fat (g)	9.5	9.5
% Fat Calories	29	26
Cholesterol (mg)	36.9	46.9
Potassium (mg)	4,643	4,880
Sodium (mg)	1,264	1,364
Omega-3 Fatty Acids (g)	1.01	1.02
Exchanges	5.4 bread/starch	5.4 bread/starch
	0 other carbs/sugar	0 other carbs/sugar
	0.7 very lean protein	0.7 very lean protein
	4.0 lean meat	4.0 lean meat
	3.4 fruit	4.5 fruit
	6.9 vegetables	6.9 vegetables
	1.7 skim milk	2.9 skim milk
	7.5 fat	7.5 fat

156

Day 21

Breakfast

1 whole wheat pita, stuffed with
    ½ cup low-fat cottage cheese
    ½ cup apricots canned in juice, drained
    2 tablespoons Spanish peanuts

Nutrition Totals 382 calories, 26.2 g protein, 48.6 g carbohydrates, 12.2 g fat

Exchanges 2.1 bread/starch, 0.3 other carbs/sugar, 2.7 very lean protein, 0.5 fruit, 1.8 fat

Morning Snack

1,500 Calories
Hot herbal tea as desired

1,800 Calories
Hot cocoa:
    1 cup skim milk, warmed
    1 packet sugar-free hot cocoa mix
    (Use milk instead of water for a
    more satisfying, richer snack.)

133 calories, 12.1 g protein,
20.4 g carbohydrates, 0.9 g fat

0.6 other carbs/sugar, 1 skim milk, 0.1 fat

Lunch

Nutty black bean salad:
    3 cups romaine lettuce
    1 cup black beans
    4 ounces canned artichoke hearts
    2 tablespoons dry-roasted sunflower seeds
    1 teaspoon olive oil
    1 tablespoon balsamic vinegar

Nutrition Totals 454 calories, 25.2 g protein, 63.1 g carbohydrates, 13.8 g fat

Exchanges 3.0 bread/starch, 0.1 other carbs/sugar, 0.3 very lean protein, 0.3 lean meat, 3.3 vegetables, 2.1 fat

Afternoon Snack

1,500 Calories
Hot cocoa:
    1 cup skim milk, warmed
    1 packet sugar-free hot cocoa mix
    (Use milk instead of water for a
    more satisfying, richer snack.)

1,800 Calories
1 serving *Ginger-Poached Pears*

133 calories, 12.1 g protein,
20.4 g carbohydrates, 0.9 g fat

0.6 other carbs/sugar, 1.0 skim milk, 0.1 fat

58 calories, 0.3 g protein,
14.9 g carbohydrates, 0.3 g fat

0.1 other carbs/sugar, 0.8 fruit

Dinner

1 serving *Creamy Pork and Parsnips*
1 kiwifruit
1 cup skim milk

Nutrition Totals 509 calories, 37.5 g protein, 71.6 g carbohydrates, 8.9 g fat

Exchanges 0.3 bread/starch, 3.4 very lean protein, 0.5 fruit, 8.6 vegetables, 0.7 skim milk, 1 fat

Evening Snack

1,500 Calories
1 serving *Ginger-Poached Pears*

58 calories, 0.3 g protein,
14.9 g carbohydrates, 0.3 g fat

0.1 other carbs/sugar, 0.8 fruit

1,800 Calories
1 serving *Fudgey Brownies*
1 cup skim milk

254 calories, 11.2 g protein,
36.2 g carbohydrates, 7.2 g fat

0.3 bread/starch, 1 other carbs/sugar,
0.2 very lean protein, 0.9 skim milk, 1.2 fat

Nutrition Totals for Day 21

	1,500 Calories	1,800 Calories
Calories	1,536	1,790
Protein (g)	101.4	112.6
Carbohydrates (g)	218.6	254.8
Fiber (g)	46.3	47.8
Fat (g)	36.1	43.3
Saturated Fat (g)	7.8	10.2
% Fat Calories	20	21
Cholesterol (mg)	97.2	101.7
Potassium (mg)	4,709	5,198
Sodium (mg)	3,071	3,282
Omega-3 Fatty Acids (g)	0.43	0.46
Exchanges	5.2 bread/starch	5.5 bread/starch
	0.9 other carbs/sugar	1.9 other carbs/sugar
	6.2 very lean protein	6.5 very lean protein
	0 lean meat	0 lean meat
	1.8 fruit	1.7 fruit
	11.8 vegetables	11.8 vegetables
	1.5 skim milk	2.4 skim milk
	4.7 fat	6.0 fat

--- **Day 22** ---

Breakfast

1 serving *Banana Chocolate Smoothie*
1 tablespoon Spanish peanuts

Nutrition Totals 375 calories, 23.1 g protein, 54.8 g carbohydrates, 9.4 g fat

Exchanges 0.2 bread/starch, 2.4 very lean protein, 1.9 fruit, 0.9 fat

Morning Snack

1,500 Calories	*1,800 Calories*
1 fresh orange	1 fresh orange
62 calories, 1.2 g protein, 15.4 g carbohydrates, 0.2 g fat	62 calories, 1.2 g protein, 15.4 g carbohydrates, 0.2 g fat
1 fruit	1 fruit

Lunch

Chickpea veggie salad:
    2 cups romaine lettuce
    ½ cup chickpeas
    5 pieces baby corn
    ½ cup grated carrots
    2 tablespoons low-fat dressing
Trail mix:
    2 tablespoons Spanish peanuts
    ¼ cup raisins

Nutrition Totals 459 calories, 21.8 g protein, 58.8 g carbohydrates, 17.9 g fat

Exchanges 1.5 bread/starch, 0.1 other carbs/sugar, 1.8 very lean protein, 1 fruit, 3.9 vegetables, 2.8 fat

Afternoon Snack

1,500 Calories	*1,800 Calories*
1 large sweet red bell pepper, sliced into strips	1 large sweet red bell pepper, sliced into strips
2 bok choy stalks	2 bok choy stalks
Dip: Mix	Dip: Mix
2 tablespoons fat-free sour cream	2 tablespoons fat-free sour cream
2 tablespoons salsa	2 tablespoons salsa

77 calories, 3.3 g protein,
16.2 g carbohydrates, 0.4 g fat

2.6 vegetables, 0.2 skim milk

77 calories, 3.3 g protein,
16.2 g carbohydrates, 0.4 g fat

2.6 vegetables, 0.2 skim milk

Dinner

1 serving *Pineapple Salmon*
1 medium baked potato with
 1 tablespoon canola margarine
1 cup fresh or frozen carrot coins, steamed
1 serving *Apricot Cream*

Nutrition Totals 548 calories, 36.6 g protein, 67.2 g carbohydrates, 15.4 g fat

Exchanges 1.4 bread/starch, 4.4 very lean protein, 1.2 fruit, 2.7 vegetables, 2.4 fat

Evening Snack

1,500 Calories
Omit

1,800 Calories
1 serving *Rich Chocolate Shake*

261 calories, 13.1 g protein,
48.2 g carbohydrates, 2.4 g fat

2.8 other carbs/sugar, 0.5 skim milk, 0.5 fat

Nutrition Totals for Day 22

	1,500 Calories	**1,800 Calories**
Calories	1,522	1,783
Protein (g)	85.9	99.1
Carbohydrates (g)	212.3	260.6
Fiber (g)	36.8	36.8
Fat (g)	43.3	45.7
Saturated Fat (g)	5.9	7.3
% Fat Calories	25	22
Cholesterol (mg)	61.7	71.8
Potassium (mg)	4,424	5,023
Sodium (mg)	965	1135
Omega-3 Fatty Acids (g)	1.76	1.77
Exchanges	3.1 bread/starch	3.1 bread/starch
	0 other carbs/sugar	2.5 other carbs/sugar
	8.6 very lean protein	8.6 very lean protein
	0 lean meat	0 lean meat
	5.0 fruit	5.0 fruit
	9.2 vegetables	9.2 vegetables
	0 skim milk	0.2 skim milk
	6.1 fat	6.6 fat

Day 23

Breakfast

1 serving *Cheesy Italian Sausage Omelet*
1 medium orange
1 slice oat bran bread, toasted

Nutrition Totals 364 calories, 32.5 g protein, 41.6 g carbohydrates, 10.6 g fat

Exchanges 1 bread/starch, 2.3 very lean protein, 1.1 lean meat, 1.2 fruit, 0.8 vegetables, 1.3 fat

Morning Snack

1,500 Calories
Omit

1,800 Calories
1 kiwifruit

50 calories, 1 g protein, 12 g carbohydrates, 0.5 g fat

0.8 fruit

Lunch

1 serving *Cream of Broccoli Soup*
1 medium apple with
    2 teaspoons peanut butter

Nutrition Totals 463 calories, 28.9 g protein, 53.6 g carbohydrates, 18.1 g fat

Exchanges 0.2 bread/starch, 1.1 very lean protein, 1 lean meat, 1.1 fruit, 3.7 vegetables, 0.5 skim milk, 2.8 fat

Afternoon Snack

1,500 Calories
1 kiwifruit

50 calories, 1 g protein,
12 g carbohydrates, 0.5 g fat

0.8 fruit

1,800 Calories
1 individual serving (8.25-ounce) "pop-top" can light peaches

120 calories, 0 protein,
30 g carbohydrates, 0 fat

1.9 fruit

Dinner

1 serving *Sage-Simmered Pork Chops*
½ cup brown rice, cooked
1 cup fresh or frozen carrot coins, steamed, with
    2 teaspoons canola margarine

1 medium pear, cored and cooked (with peel), dipped in
2 teaspoons brown Sugar Twin
1 tablespoon fat-free sour cream

Nutrition Totals 574 calories, 29.9 g protein, 74 g carbohydrates, 18.8 g fat

Exchanges 1.7 bread/starch, 3 very lean protein, 1.5 fruit, 3.3 vegetables, 2.9 fat

Evening Snack

1,500 Calories
1 individual serving (8.25-ounce) "pop-top" can light peaches

120 calories, 0 protein,
30 g carbohydrates, 0 fat

1.9 fruit

1,800 Calories
1 serving *Double Raspberry Shake*

205 calories, 9.4 g protein,
41.8 g carbohydrates, 0.6 g fat

1.5 other carbs/sugar, 0.5 fruit, 1 skim milk

Nutrition Totals for Day 23

	1,500 Calories	1,800 Calories
Calories	1,567	1,772
Protein (g)	92	101.4
Carbohydrates (g)	210.6	252.4
Fiber (g)	44	45.8
Fat (g)	47.9	48.5
Saturated Fat (g)	13.6	13.8
% Fat Calories	26	24
Cholesterol (mg)	96.8	101.1
Potassium (mg)	3,051	3,642
Sodium (mg)	2,285	2,421
Omega-3 Fatty Acids (g)	0.77	0.77
Exchanges	2.9 bread/starch	2.9 bread/starch
	0 other carbs/sugar	1.1 other carbs/sugar
	6.4 very lean protein	6.4 very lean protein
	1.9 lean meat	1.9 lean meat
	6.4 fruit	6.8 fruit
	7.8 vegetables	7.8 vegetables
	0.4 skim milk	1.4 skim milk
	7.0 fat	7.0 fat

Day 24

Breakfast

3 servings *The Moistest Zucchini-Carrot Muffins*
1 cup skim milk

Nutrition Totals 341 calories, 15.5 g protein, 42.7 g carbohydrates, 12.9 g fat

Exchanges 1.1 bread/starch, 0.5 other carbs/sugar, 0.4 very lean protein, 0.2 lean meat, 0.1 fruit, 0.4 vegetables, 0.9 skim milk, 2.2 fat

Morning Snack

1,500 Calories
Omit

1,800 Calories
1 fresh papaya

119 calories, 1.8 g protein, 29.8 g carbohydrates, 0.4 g fat

2.1 fruit

Lunch

1 serving *Cheddar Cheese Potato Leek Soup*
Sun-dried tomato salad:
      3 cups spinach
      ¼ cup sun-dried tomatoes
      Favorite flavored vinegar
      1 teaspoon freshly ground black pepper
1 cup skim milk

Nutrition Totals 448 calories, 30.5 g protein, 66 g carbohydrates, 10.2 g fat

Exchanges 1 bread/starch, 0.1 other carbs/sugar, 1.2 lean meat, 5 vegetables, 1.5 skim milk, 1.1 fat

Afternoon Snack

1,500 Calories
1 serving *Zesty Cauliflower Salad*

98 calories, 4 g protein, 13.1 g carbohydrates, 3.9 g fat

0.2 bread/starch, 0.2 other carbs/sugar, 1.7 vegetables, 0.7 fat

1,800 Calories
1 serving *Zesty Cauliflower Salad*

98 calories, 4 g protein, 13.1 g carbohydrates, 3.9 g fat

0.2 bread/starch, 0.2 other carbs/sugar, 1.7 vegetables, 0.7 fat

Dinner

1 serving *Herbed Chicken and Pasta*
1 cup fresh or frozen strawberries

Nutrition Totals 515 calories, 38.7 g protein, 54.7 g carbohydrates, 15.6 g fat

Exchanges 1.8 bread/starch, 3.5 very lean protein, 0.8 fruit, 2.6 vegetables, 2.3 fat

Evening Snack

1,500 Calories
1 fresh papaya

119 calories, 1.8 g protein,
29.8 g carbohydrates, 0.4 g fat

2.1 fruit

1,800 Calories
1 serving *Raspberry Cream Gelatin*,
topped with 2 tablespoons dry-roasted
almonds

278 calories, 22 g protein,
26.7 g carbohydrates, 9.5 g fat

0.3 bread/starch, 1 other carbs/sugar,
2.3 very lean protein, 0.3 lean meat,
0.5 fruit, 1.2 fat

Nutrition Totals for Day 24

	1,500 Calories	**1,800 Calories**
Calories	1,520	1,797
Protein (g)	90.5	112.5
Carbohydrates (g)	206.4	233
Fiber (g)	32.1	38.3
Fat (g)	43	52.4
Saturated Fat (g)	9.4	10.2
% Fat Calories	25	25
Cholesterol (mg)	111	117.1
Potassium (mg)	5,237	5,534
Sodium (mg)	2,805	3,455
Omega-3 Fatty Acids (g)	1.90	2.02
Exchanges	4.0 bread/starch	4.3 bread/starch
	0.2 other carbs/sugar	1.2 other carbs/sugar
	3.4 very lean protein	5.7 very lean protein
	0.6 lean meat	0.8 lean meat
	2.8 fruit	3.3 fruit
	9.7 vegetables	9.6 vegetables
	1.6 skim milk	1.4 skim milk
	6.2 fat	7.4 fat

Day 25

Breakfast

1 serving *Kris's Highest Fiber (and Moistest) Bread* with 2 tablespoons roasted soy butter
1 cup skim milk

Nutrition Totals 395 calories, 20.5 g protein, 43.9 g carbohydrates, 15.8 g fat

Exchanges 1.8 bread/starch, 0.1 other carbs/sugar, 0.1 very lean protein, 0.9 lean meat, 1 skim milk, 2.3 fat

Morning Snack

1,500 Calories
Omit

1,800 Calories
4 bok choy stalks
1 cup raw broccoli florets
2 tablespoons salsa

36 calories, 3.4 g protein, 7 g carbohydrates, 0.4 g fat

1.4 vegetables

Lunch

Salad-stuffed pita:
    1 whole wheat pita pocket
    ½ cup black beans (boiled or canned)
    1 carrot, grated
    6 cherry tomatoes, quartered
    2 cups spinach
    1 tablespoon olive oil

Nutrition Totals 468 calories, 17 g protein, 68 g carbohydrates, 16.8 g fat

Exchanges 3.5 bread/starch, 0.2 very lean protein, 2.4 vegetables, 2.8 fat

Afternoon Snack

1,500 Calories
1 banana

109 calories, 1.2 g protein, 27.6 g carbohydrates, 0.6 g fat

1.9 fruit

1,800 Calories
1 fresh papaya
½ cup low-fat frozen yogurt

220 calories, 6.3 g protein, 48.3 g carbohydrates, 1.7g fat

1.3 other carbs/sugar, 2.1 fruit, 0.3 fat

Dinner

1 serving *Sweet-and-Sour Tuna*
½ cup medium-grain brown rice
4 large fresh or frozen broccoli spears, steamed, spritzed with
    lemon juice as desired

Nutrition Totals 510 calories, 47.5 g protein, 57.7 g carbohydrates, 10 g fat

Exchanges 1.6 bread/starch, 5.4 very lean protein, 0.9 fruit, 3.2 vegetables, 1.3 fat

Evening Snack

1,500 Calories
1 kiwifruit

1,800 Calories
1 Snackwell's Fat-Free Devil's Food
    Cookie
1½ cups skim milk

46 calories, 0.8 g protein,
11.3 g carbohydrates, 0.3 g fat

0.8 fruit

168 calories, 12.4 g protein,
28.4 g carbohydrates, 0.8 g fat

0.7 other carbs/sugar, 1.4 skim milk

Nutrition Totals for Day 25

	1,500 Calories	**1,800 Calories**
Calories	1,528	1,797
Protein (g)	87	107.1
Carbohydrates (g)	208.5	253.2
Fiber (g)	36.4	39.8
Fat (g)	43.5	45.6
Saturated Fat (g)	6.4	7.7
% Fat Calories	25	22
Cholesterol (mg)	90	101.2
Potassium (mg)	4,105	5,385
Sodium (mg)	1,595	2,057
Omega-3 Fatty Acids (g)	1.53	1.67
Exchanges	6.9 bread/starch	6.9 bread/starch
	0 other carbs/sugar	1.6 other carbs/sugar
	5.6 very lean protein	5.6 very lean protein
	0.4 lean meat	0.4 lean meat
	3.5 fruit	3.0 fruit
	5.6 vegetables	7.0 vegetables
	0.5 skim milk	1.8 skim milk
	6.5 fat	6.8 fat

Day 26

Breakfast

1 serving *Peanut Butter Chocolate Smoothie*
1 medium banana

Nutrition Totals 365 calories, 15.6 g protein, 54.7 g carbohydrates, 11.9 g fat

Exchanges 0.1 bread/starch, 0.8 very lean protein, 0.4 lean meat, 1.9 fruit, 2.2 skim milk, 1.6 fat

Morning Snack

1,500 Calories
Omit

1,800 Calories
1 fresh orange

64 calories, 2.1 g protein,
24.6 g carbohydrates, 0.5 g fat

1.6 fruit

Lunch

1 serving *Fresh Vegetable and Lentil Salad*
½ cup skim milk

Nutrition Totals 450 calories, 26 g protein, 68.5 g carbohydrates, 12.1 g fat

Exchanges 2.4 bread/starch, 0.2 very lean protein, 0.3 lean meat, 4.9 vegetables, 0.5 skim milk, 1.6 fat

Afternoon Snack

1,500 Calories
1 fresh orange

1,800 Calories
1 cup raw cauliflower
10 raw snow peas
5 cherry tomatoes
Dip: Blend
      2 tablespoons reduced-fat
      sour cream
      3 fresh basil leaves,
      finely chopped

64 calories, 2.1 g protein,
24.6 g carbohydrates, 0.5 g fat

1.6 fruit

105 calories, 5.1 g protein,
13.8 g carbohydrates, 4.3 g fat

0.2 bread/starch, 1.8 vegetables,
0.2 skim milk, 0.7 fat

167

Dinner

1 serving *Beef Stew*
½ cup barley, cooked
1 serving *Ginger-Poached Pears*

Nutrition Totals 546 calories, 36.1 g protein, 70.6 g carbohydrates, 11.5 g fat

Exchanges 2.2 bread/starch, 4.3 very lean protein, 0.6 fruit, 1.7 vegetables, 1.6 fat

Evening Snack

1,500 Calories
1 cup raw cauliflower
10 raw snow peas
5 cherry tomatoes
Dip: Blend
     2 tablespoons reduced-fat
     sour cream
     3 fresh basil leaves,
     finely chopped

105 calories, 5.1 g protein,
13.8 g carbohydrates, 4.3 g fat

0.2 bread/starch, 1.8 vegetables,
0.2 skim milk, 0.7 fat

1,800 Calories
6 Hershey's Chocolate Kisses
1 cup skim milk

231 calories, 10.3 g protein,
28.7 g carbohydrates, 9.1 g fat

1.1 other carbs/sugar, 1 skim milk, 1.5 fat

Nutrition Totals for Day 26

	1,500 Calories	**1,800 Calories**
Calories	1,529	1,760
Protein (g)	88.3	98.6
Carbohydrates (g)	232.2	260.9
Fiber (g)	46.3	47.2
Fat (g)	40.3	49.5
Saturated Fat (g)	10	15.5
% Fat Calories	22	24
Cholesterol (mg)	112.8	123.4
Potassium (mg)	5,406	5,921
Sodium (mg)	948	1,098
Omega-3 Fatty Acids (g)	1.81	1.81
Exchanges	4.9 bread/starch	4.9 bread/starch
	0 other carbs/sugar	1.0 other carbs/sugar
	5.2 very lean protein	5.2 very lean protein
	0.2 lean meat	0.2 lean meat
	4.1 fruit	4.1 fruit
	8.3 vegetables	8.3 vegetables
	2.4 skim milk	3.3 skim milk
	5.5 fat	7.0 fat

Day 27

Breakfast

3 *Blueberry Muffins*
½ cup skim milk

Nutrition Totals 356 calories, 16.5 g protein, 53.6 g carbohydrates, 9.8 g fat

Exchanges 1.9 bread/starch, 0.4 other carbs/sugar, 0.3 very lean protein, 0.5 fruit, 0.6 skim milk, 1.7 fat

Morning Snack

1,500 Calories
Omit

1,800 Calories
1 banana

109 calories, 1.2 g protein, 27.6 g carbohydrates, 0.6 g fat

1.9 fruit

Lunch

Ham and cheese sandwich:
    2 slices whole wheat bread
    2 ounces extra-lean sliced ham
    1 slice low-fat cheddar cheese
    1 tablespoon light mayonnaise or light Miracle Whip
10 baby carrots
1 fresh apple

Nutrition Totals 431 calories, 24.5 g protein, 57.4 g carbohydrates, 13.1 g fat

Exchanges 1.7 bread/starch, 0.1 other carbs/sugar, 2.6 very lean protein, 1.4 fruit, 1.6 vegetables, 1.9 fat

Afternoon Snack

1,500 Calories
1 fresh orange

69 calories, 1.1 g protein, 17.4 g carbohydrates, 0.3 g fat

1.2 fruit

1,800 Calories
1 serving *Lemon Torte*

138 calories, 5.4 g protein, 26.6 g carbohydrates, 1.1 g fat

0.7 bread/starch, 0.8 other carbs/sugar, 0.5 very lean protein

Dinner

1 serving *Pasta Primavera with Spinach Noodles*
Carrot-romaine salad:
>   2 cups romaine lettuce
>   1 carrot, grated
>   ¼ cup seasoned croutons
>   2 tablespoons favorite light salad dressing

Nutrition Totals 525 calories, 24.1 g protein, 73.1 g carbohydrates, 16.8 g fat

Exchanges 3.1 bread/starch, 3.9 vegetables, 2.4 fat

Evening Snack

1,500 Calories
1 serving *Lemon Torte*

138 calories, 5.4 g protein,
26.6 g carbohydrates, 1.1 g fat

0.7 bread/starch, 0.8 other carbs/
sugar, 0.5 very lean protein

1,800 Calories
1 serving *Berry Fresh Cheesecake*

222 calories, 15.6 g protein,
26.4 g carbohydrates, 5.6 g fat

0.4 bread/starch, 0.7 other carbs/sugar,
1.7 very lean protein, 0.4 lean meat,
0.2 fruit, 0.9 fat

Nutrition Totals for Day 27

	1,500 Calories	1,800 Calories
Calories	1,519	1,781
Protein (g)	71.6	87.3
Carbohydrates (g)	228.2	264.7
Fiber (g)	37	38.3
Fat (g)	41.1	46.9
Saturated Fat (g)	7.6	11.2
% Fat Calories	24	23
Cholesterol (mg)	90.5	111.1
Potassium (mg)	3,536	4,010
Sodium (mg)	2,766	3,284
Omega-3 Fatty Acids (g)	0.70	0.83
Exchanges	7.5 bread/starch	8.0 bread/starch
	1.3 other carbs/sugar	2.0 other carbs/sugar
	3.4 very lean protein	5.1 very lean protein
	0 lean meat	0 lean meat
	3.1 fruit	4.1 fruit
	5.2 vegetables	5.1 vegetables
	0.2 skim milk	0.1 skim milk
	5.8 fat	6.7 fat

Day 28

Breakfast

1 packet instant oatmeal, reconstituted with
    ¾ cup low-fat fortified soy milk, warmed
    2 tablespoons sliced almonds
1 fresh orange

Nutrition Totals 366 calories, 16.6 g protein, 46.6 g carbohydrates, 13.5 g fat

Exchanges 1.9 bread/starch, 1.3 lean meat, 1 fruit, 1.8 fat

Morning Snack

1,500 Calories	*1,800 Calories*
Omit	1 fresh apple
	81 calories, 0.3 g protein, 21.0 g carbohydrates, 0.5 g fat
	1.4 fruit

Lunch

Grilled cheese sandwich (spray pan with vegetable oil and grill):
    2 slices *Kris's Highest Fiber (and Moistest) Bread*
    2 slices soy cheese
    ½ medium tomato, sliced
1 cup skim milk

Nutrition Totals 454 calories, 27.3 g protein, 58.8 g carbohydrates, 12.8 g fat

Exchanges 2.1 bread/starch, 0.3 other carbs/sugar, 0.1 very lean protein, 0.4 lean meat, 2.1 vegetables, 0.9 skim milk, 2.1 fat

Afternoon Snack

1,500 Calories	*1,800 Calories*
1 medium apple	1 serving *Apricot Cream*
81 calories, 0.3 g protein, 21.0 g carbohydrates, 0.5 g fat	88 calories, 10.5 g protein, 11.5 g carbohydrates, 0.2 g fat
1.4 fruit	1.3 very lean protein, 0.6 fruit

Dinner

1 serving *Grilled Beef Fajitas*
1 cup mandarin orange sections

Salad:
>   2 cups romaine lettuce
>   4 ounces artichoke hearts
>   ¼ cup grated carrots

Olive-lemon dressing:
>   1 teaspoon olive oil
>   1 tablespoon balsamic vinegar
>   1 teaspoon lemon juice

Nutrition Totals 536 calories, 29.9 g protein, 72.3 g carbohydrates, 16.4 g fat

Exchanges 1.1 bread/starch, 0.3 other carbs/sugar, 2.5 lean meat, 0.9 fruit, 5.5 vegetables, 0.1 skim milk, 1.6 fat

Evening Snack

1,500 Calories
1 serving *Apricot Cream*

88 calories, 10.5 g protein, 11.5 g carbohydrates, 0.2 g fat

1.3 very lean protein, 0.6 fruit

1,800 Calories
1 serving *Fudgey Brownies*
1 cup skim milk

254 calories, 11.2 g protein, 36.2 g carbohydrates, 7.2 g fat

0.3 bread/starch, 1 other carbs/sugar, 0.2 very lean protein, 0.9 skim milk, 1.2 fat

Nutrition Totals for Day 28

	1,500 Calories	**1,800 Calories**
Calories	1,526	1,780
Protein (g)	84.6	95.9
Carbohydrates (g)	210.3	246.5
Fiber (g)	34.6	36.1
Fat (g)	43.4	50.6
Saturated Fat (g)	6.1	8.5
% Fat Calories	25	25
Cholesterol (mg)	64.9	69.4
Potassium (mg)	3,441	3,930
Sodium (mg)	1,975	2,186
Omega-3 Fatty Acids (g)	0.33	0.36
Exchanges	4.9 bread/starch	5.2 bread/starch
	0.4 other carbs/sugar	1.5 other carbs/sugar
	0.9 very lean protein	1.2 very lean protein
	4.1 lean meat	4.0 lean meat
	3.8 fruit	3.8 fruit
	7.4 vegetables	7.4 vegetables
	0.9 skim milk	1.8 skim milk
	5.4 fat	6.6 fat

Chapter Nine

Nutrient Roundup

In years gone by, the common term to describe nutrient requirements was Recommended Dietary Allowance (RDA). Today, all that is changing as research advances and nutrition scientists learn more about the body's needs for and use of nutrients, both in preventing nutrient deficiencies and also in preventing chronic disease. The new term is Dietary Reference Intake (DRI), which refers to at least three types of reference values. These are the terms that you need to help read the following charts.

- Estimated Average Requirement: Intake value that is estimated to meet the requirement defined by a specified indicator of adequacy in 50% of an age- and gender-specific group. At this level of intake, the remaining 50 percent of the specified group would not have its needs met.

- Recommended Dietary Allowance: Dietary intake level sufficient to meet the nutrient requirements of nearly all individuals in the group.

- Tolerable Upper Intake Level: Maximum level of daily nutrient intake unlikely to pose risks of adverse health effects to almost all of the individuals in the group for whom it is designed.

Vitamins

Nutrient	Recommended Daily Intake	Why We Need It	Adverse Effects if Taken in Excess	Recommended Foods
Vitamin A (Retinol)	RDA: Men: 900 mcg Women: 700 mcg	• Essential for vision • Enhances immunity • Builds and maintains bone	Headache Vomiting Blurred vision Liver damage Birth defects	Orange fruits Leafy green vegetables
Vitamin B$_1$ (Thiamin)	RDA: Men (19 and over): 1.2 mg Women (19 and over): 1.1 mg	• Releases energy from carbohydrates, protein, and fat • Essential for nerve function	Not toxic if taken orally	Yeast Legumes Seeds Nuts Unrefined cereal
Vitamin B$_2$ (Riboflavin)	RDA: Men (19 and over): 1.3 mg Women (19 and over): 1.1 mg	• Releases energy from carbohydrates, protein, and fat • An ingredient in hormones • Prevents anemia • May prevent migraine headache at higher doses	Not toxic	Skim milk Leafy green vegetables Whole grain bread Skim milk or low-fat yogurt Skim or 1% fat cottage cheese Meat
Vitamin B$_3$ (Niacin)	RDA: Men: 16 mg Women: 14 mg	• Releases energy from carbohydrates, protein, and fat • Helps prevent anemia	Upper limit of safe intake: 35 mg Flushing Liver problems Aggravates asthma Ulcers Glucose intolerance associated with Type 2 diabetes	Legumes Nuts Whole grain bread Fish Meat

Nutrient	Recommended Daily Intake	Why We Need It	Adverse Effects if Taken in Excess	Recommended Foods
Vitamin B$_6$ (Pyridoxine)	RDA: Men (19–50): 1.3 mg Women (19–50): 1.3 mg Men (51 and over): 1.7 mg Women (51 and over): 1.5 mg	• Helps break down protein • Essential for healthy nerve function • May prevent high blood cholesterol and heart disease • May prevent depression • May ensure clear thinking later in life	Prolonged use of more than 250 mg per day can cause sensitivity to light and irreversible neurological symptoms	Bananas Many vegetables, including peas, potatoes, sweet potatoes Chicken (skinless) Fish Lean pork
Biotin	AI: 30 mcg	• Necessary for energy reactions • Makes fatty acids • Breaks down amino acids	Not toxic at doses up to 10 mg	Soybeans and soy products Yeast
Folate (Folic Acid, Folacin)	RDA: 400 mcg	• Helps make new cells • Prevents anemia • Prevents some birth defects • May prevent high blood cholesterol, heart disease, cancer, and depression • May ensure clear thinking in later life	Upper limit of safe intake: 1,000 mcg At levels greater than 1 mg: Masks the symptoms of B$_{12}$ deficiency and pernicious anemia	Yeast Leafy green vegetables such as spinach, romaine lettuce, mustard greens, and many others Fruits such as oranges, bananas, papayas Legumes such as lentils, black beans, and many more
Vitamin B$_{12}$ (Cobalamin)	RDA: 2.4 mcg	• Helps make new cells • Maintains healthy nerve fibers • May prevent high cholesterol and heart disease • May prevent depression	Not toxic up to 100 mcg	Clams Oysters Skim milk Seafood Egg whites Fortified soy milk Fish and lean meat

(continued)

Nutrient	Recommended Daily Intake	Why We Need It	Adverse Effects if Taken in Excess	Recommended Foods
Pantothenic Acid	AI: 5 mg	• Necessary to make fatty acids	None known	Whole grains Legumes Mushrooms Avocado Broccoli Yeast
Vitamin C (Ascorbic Acid)	Men: 90 mg Women: 75 mg Up to 100 mg for smokers. People under stress, who have undergone surgery, or who have Type 2 diabetes may have higher requirements.	• Acts as extracellular antioxidant • Helps form essential hormones • Recycles vitamin E as an antioxidant • May prevent atherosclerotic heart disease when obtained through food but not high-dose supplements	Nausea and diarrhea May decrease copper levels Reduces serum levels of B_{12} Inhibits utilization of beta-carotene May increase risk of atherosclerosis when taken in high-dose supplements	Citrus fruits Nearly all vegetables, but especially green vegetables, peppers, and tomatoes Berries Potatoes
Vitamin D	Less than 50 years of age: 5 mcg Over 50 years of age: 10 mcg	• Helps absorb calcium • Essential component of hormones	Leaches calcium from bones and teeth Kidney damage Artery hardening Death	Sunlight, if you do not wear sunscreen, if you do not have dark skin, and are under age 60 Fattier fish such as salmon and mackerel Skim milk Fortified soy milk

Nutrient	Recommended Daily Intake	Why We Need It	Adverse Effects if Taken in Excess	Recommended Foods
Vitamin E (Tocopherol)	15 mg	• Prevents anemia and neurological abnormalities as an antioxidant • Helps protect cells from damage caused by oxygen-free radicals	Gastrointestinal discomfort Impaired immune function Flu-like symptoms	Vegetable oils Wheat germ Nuts Green leafy vegetables Many fruits and vegetables (see list in Chapter Six)
Vitamin K	Men: 120 mcg Women: 90 mcg	• Necessary for normal blood clotting • May be needed for building bone	None known	Green leafy vegetables Milk Cabbage Soybean oil

Minerals

Nutrient	Recommended Daily Intake	Why We Need It	Adverse Effects if Taken in Excess	Recommended Foods
Arsenic	Undetermined	• Needed for growth and optimal iron use	Quickly toxic at higher than recommended doses	Fish Grain Cereal products
Boron	Undetermined	• Necessary for healthy cell membranes and hormone function	Vomiting Diarrhea Fatigue Encourages loss of riboflavin through the urine	Leafy vegetables Nuts Legumes Non-citrus fruits
Calcium	AI: Ages 31–50: 1,000 mg Older than 51: 1,200 mg	• Essential in forming bones • May lower blood pressure and prevent colon cancer	Upper limit of safe intake for adults older than age 19: 2,500 Inhibits absorption of other minerals, especially iron and magnesium (take calcium, iron, and magnesium supplements at different times of day) Increases vitamin C metabolism, causing loss of vitamin Causes kidney stones, fatigue, muscle weakness, depression, anorexia, nausea	Nonfat milk and dairy products Green leafy vegetables Sardines Salmon, especially canned pink salmon with bones Low-fat tofu Fortified soy milk

Nutrient	Recommended Daily Intake	Why We Need It	Adverse Effects if Taken in Excess	Recommended Foods
Chloride	Undetermined	• Fluid balance • Essential ingredient in stomach acid	Elevated blood pressure	Dietary salt and salt substitutes containing chloride, such as potassium chloride
Chromium	Safe and adequate intake: Men (19–50): 35 mcg Women (19–50): 25 mcg Men (51 and over): 30 mcg Women (51 and over): 20 mcg	• Helps metabolize carbohydrates and fats • Essential for insulin to work properly	Decreases zinc absorption	Mushrooms Prunes Nuts Asparagus Some lean meats Whole grains Cheese
Cobalt	There is no evidence that the intake of cobalt is ever lacking in the human diet, and no RDA is necessary.	• Important ingredient of vitamin B_{12}	May interfere with iron absorption	Foods rich in B_{12} such as meat and milk
Copper	RDA: 900 mcg	• Essential for using iron, making connective tissue, and forming energy	Decreases zinc and iron absorption Increases metabolism of riboflavin and B_6, which are then lost from the body	Legumes Seafood and shellfish Whole grains Nuts Seeds Vegetables
Fluoride	AI: Men: 4 mcg Women: 3 mcg	• Increases hardness of bones and teeth	Fluorosis, or mottling of teeth	Fluoridated water
Iodine	RDA: 150 mcg	• Makes thyroid hormones	Intakes up to 2 mg apparently not dangerous	Iodized salt Dairy products

(continued)

Nutrient	Recommended Daily Intake	Why We Need It	Adverse Effects if Taken in Excess	Recommended Foods
Iron	RDA: Men: 8 mg Women: age 19–50: 18 mcg 51 and over: 8 mcg	• Prevents anemia	Iron overload can damage the pancreas, liver, and heart Reduces copper levels Interferes with zinc and calcium absorption (take these supplements at different times of day) Increases metabolism of B$_{12}$, riboflavin, niacin, and folate	Lean meats Fish Poultry Organ meats Legumes Nuts and seeds Whole grains Dark molasses Green leafy vegetables
Magnesium	RDA: Men: 420 mg Women: 320 mg	• Necessary for absorbing and using calcium • May help control blood pressure	Increases metabolism of thiamin, vitamin C, vitamin B$_6$, causing loss from the body	Unprocessed whole grains (80% of magnesium is lost during processing of whole grains into refined products) Legumes Nuts and seeds Chocolate Dark green vegetables Bananas
Manganese	Safe and adequate intake: 2 to 5 mg	• Helps make many enzymes • Needed for energy reactions	Toxicity from dietary intake is rare but affects the brain when it does occur Decreases magnesium absorption Increases metabolism of riboflavin, niacin, and thiamin, causing loss of these nutrients	Whole grain cereal products Many fruits and vegetables Many legumes Tea

Nutrient	Recommended Daily Intake	Why We Need It	Adverse Effects if Taken in Excess	Recommended Foods
Molybdenum	Safe and adequate intake: Men: 45 mcg Women: 45 mcg	• Helps to produce energy		Milk Beans Breads Cereals
Nickel	Undetermined	• Not entirely understood, but probably an ingredient in a number of enzymes	Gastrointestinal irritation	Chocolate Nuts Dried beans and peas Grains
Phosphorus	RDA: 700 mg	• Necessary for forming cells essential to metabolism of carbohydrates, protein, and fat • Helps transport fat in bloodstream; moves nutrients into and out of cells	Causes bone loss Interferes with calcium absorption	Many fruits and vegetables Cereal grains Skim milk Nonfat milk products Lean meat
Potassium	Undetermined	• Essential for proper muscle function • Regulates heartbeat	Causes irregular heartbeat and cardiac arrest	Fruits Vegetables Legumes Meat
Selenium	RDA: 55 mcg	• Functions as antioxidant	Damages nervous system Causes skin lesions, thicker but more fragile nails, loss of hair and nails, nausea, abdominal pain, diarrhea, fatigue, irritability Interferes with antioxidant balance of cell Increases copper metabolism, causing copper to be lost from the body	Brazil nuts (did you know that 1 Brazil nut gives you all the selenium you need for the day!) Seafood Lean meat Egg whites Whole grains Legumes

(continued)

Nutrient	Recommended Daily Intake	Why We Need It	Adverse Effects if Taken in Excess	Recommended Foods
Silicon	Undetermined	• Helps form connective tissue, necessary for making strong bones	None known	Unrefined grains with high fiber content Root vegetables such as potatoes, carrots, parsnips, and others
Sodium	Undetermined	• Regulates fluid balance in body • Helps in metabolism of carbohydrates and protein	Causes fluid retention and hypertension in some people Leaches calcium from bones	Processed foods
Vanadium	Undetermined	• Thought to regulate enzyme and hormone functions	May cause gastrointestinal problems such as cramps and diarrhea	Shellfish Mushrooms Parsley Black pepper
Zinc	RDA: Men (19 and over): 11 mg Women (19 and over): 8 mg	• Necessary for growth, immune function, blood clotting, wound healing	Lowers HDL (good) cholesterol and levels of copper Shrinks red blood cells, decreasing amount of oxygen they carry Impairs immunity Increases metabolism of niacin, B_6, vitamin E, and vitamin A, causing loss of these nutrients in body	Lean meat Eggs Seafood Nuts Whole grains

Aluminum, tin, cadmium, lead, germanium, lithium, and rubidium have all been studied, but there is insufficient evidence that they are essential to human health.

Daily Values

Nutrition Panel Format

All nutrients must be declared as percentages of the Daily Values, which are label reference values. The amount, in grams or milligrams, of macronutrients (such as fat, cholesterol, sodium, carbohydrates, and protein) is listed to the immediate right of these nutrients. A column headed "% Daily Value" appears on the far right side.

There are several reasons why Daily Value (DV) is not useful. Most importantly, DV is based on antiquated recommended dietary allowances, most of which have been updated.

While declaring nutrients as a percentage of the Daily Values is intended to prevent misinterpretations that arise with quantitative values, many times they have the opposite impact. For example, a food with 140 milligrams of sodium could be mistaken for a high-sodium food because 140 is a relatively large number. In actuality, however, that amount represents less than 6 percent of the Daily Value for sodium, which is 2,400 milligrams.

On the other hand, a food with 5 grams of saturated fat could be construed as being low in that nutrient. In fact, that food would provide one-fourth of the total Daily Value because 20 grams is the Daily Value for saturated fat.

Nutrition Panel Footnote

The % Daily Value listing carries a footnote saying that the percentages are based on a 2,000-calorie diet. Some nutrition labels—at least those on larger packages—have these additional notes:

- A sentence that indicates a person's individual nutrient goals are based on his or her calorie needs (basically telling you to ignore DV).
- Lists of the daily values for selected nutrients for diets of 2,000 and 2,500 calories (more calories than most adults need).

Reference Values for Nutrition Labeling

Nutrition labels tell you which nutrients are contained in a particular food. One column on a nutrition label has "% of DV"—in other words, it shows what percentage of the Daily Value you're getting from that particular food. The information on those labels is based upon the following table, which indicates the recommended intake for adults and for children over the age of four who have 2,000 calories in their daily diet. For many reasons (see page 183), these values are probably not ideal for you, especially if you're eating less than 2,000 calories every day. However, this chart helps to show you the range of nutrients, how they are measured, and what the food industry is using (as of 1999) to calculate "% of DV" that's shown on labels.

Nutrient	Unit of Measure	Daily Values
Total Fat	Gram (g)	65
Saturated Fatty Acids	Gram (g)	20
Cholesterol	Milligram (mg)	300
Sodium	Milligram (mg)	2,400
Potassium	Milligram (mg)	3,500
Total Carbohydrate	Gram (g)	300
Fiber	Gram (g)	25
Protein	Gram (g)	50
Vitamin A	International Unit (IU)	5,000
Vitamin C	Milligram (mg)	60
Calcium	Milligram (mg)	1,000
Iron	Milligram (mg)	18
Vitamin D	International Unit (IU)	400
Vitamin E	International Unit (IU)	30
Vitamin K	Microgram (μg)	80

Nutrient Roundup

Nutrient	Unit of Measure	Daily Values
Thiamin	Milligram (mg)	1.5
Riboflavin	Milligram (mg)	1.7
Niacin	Milligram (mg)	20
Vitamin B_6	Milligram (mg)	2.0
Folate	Microgram (µg)	400
Vitamin B_{12}	Microgram (µg)	6.0
Biotin	Microgram (µg)	300
Pantothenic Acid	Milligram (mg)	10
Phosphorus	Milligram (mg)	1,000
Iodine	Microgram (µg)	150
Magnesium	Milligram (mg)	400
Zinc	Milligram (mg)	15
Selenium	Microgram (µg)	70
Copper	Milligram (mg)	2.0
Manganese	Milligram (mg)	2.0
Chromium	Microgram (µg)	120
Molybdenum	Microgram (µg)	75
Chloride	Milligram (mg)	3,400

Source: U.S. Food and Drug Administration, Center for Food Safety and Applied Nutrition, September 1994 (editorial revisions June 1999).

Chapter Ten

What About Chromium, Vitamin E, and Other Supplements?

Should you take one single vitamin supplement containing all nutrients or many pills containing one nutrient each? Or is the answer no supplements at all but just the right combination of foods? No doubt you've asked these questions about nutrient supplements. And perhaps, to be on the safe side, you pop one or a combination of nutrient supplements, from vitamin A to the herb valerian.

This chapter will help you understand the debate that continues about various supplements that have been recommended over time for people with diabetes as well as some popular ones recommended for heart disease and other common conditions. Because this particular topic is at once intriguing and confusing, I am going to give you the bottom line on vitamins and minerals, and then fill in the details.

Magnesium: There is no conclusive evidence that people with diabetes will benefit from supplementation over the recommended intake; *however, it is very important that you do get adequate intakes of magnesium through an eating plan that supplies sufficient amounts.*

Chromium: There is no conclusive evidence that you will benefit from supplementation over the recommended intake, *but as with magnesium, it is important to harvest an adequate intake through a nutrient-rich diet.*

Zinc: While zinc also plays a quintessential role in energy metabolism, experts do not yet recommend supplements. This is one area where I recommend a slightly higher intake.

Vitamin E: While the most recent evidence found that vitamin E does not reduce heart disease risk in the general population, there is some evidence that vitamin E supplementation may help reduce death from heart disease in people with diabetes. There may be some benefit to taking 400 IU per day of synthetic vitamin E or 200 IU per day of natural vitamin E. Always check with your physician about any supplements you plan to take or are taking.

Getting Extra Versus Enough

Today, we all demand quick fixes. We all look for the pill that will bring us good health, prevent disease, and, if we're diabetic, improve blood sugars. The truth is, there just isn't any convincing research that taking excessive amounts of any one nutrient will help with any of these things. You should note, however, that taking excessive amounts is distinctly different from getting the amount you need—which is definitely recommended!

Magnesium

The reason that magnesium comes up so often in the context of diabetes is that one of its roles in the body is to aid in the use and storage of glucose. Indeed, without adequate amounts of magnesium, the body does not metabolize glucose efficiently. The body also needs magnesium for using and storing—that is, metabolizing—amino acids and fatty acids.

In addition to its role in metabolism, magnesium is an essential ingredient and instigator in several other body processes:

- Helping the heart beat normally
- Preventing heart attacks
- Maintaining normal muscle contraction
- Ensuring normal nerve function
- Building strong bones, with the help of calcium and phosphorus
- Possibly preventing kidney stones
- Spurring countless chemical, hormonal, and enzymatic reactions: Magnesium is a co-factor in more than three hundred biochemical reactions, many of which involve the use or formation of adenosine triphosphate (ATP), the energy currency of the body.

But let's go back to the question of whether or not getting extra magnesium can help you metabolize glucose better. The answer is probably no. That said, however, it is imperative to take in the recommended amount of magnesium for good health. Not getting the recommended amount of magnesium can cause problems with insulin resistance. But getting enough magnesium and other minerals is difficult for many Americans, especially those who do not eat enough vegetables, whole grains, and legumes. The following chart lists how much magnesium you need every day as well as some good sources of this quintessential mineral.

Recommended Dietary Allowance
Men: 420 mg per day
Women: 320 mg per day

MAGNESIUM

Food	Amount	Milligrams
All-Bran cereal	1 cup	207.4
Almonds, slivered	¼ cup	100.0
Amaranth	¼ cup	129.6
Avocado	1 each	103.0
Baked potato with skin	1 each	32.9
Banana	1 each	33.1

(continued)

189

Food	Amount	Milligrams
Barley, cooked	1 cup	44.4
Black beans, cooked	1 cup	120.0
Black walnuts	¼ cup	63.3
Blueberry waffle	2	16.2
Brewer's yeast	2 tablespoons	37.0
Broad beans (fava beans), cooked	1 cup	73.1
Bulgur, cooked	⅝ cup	57.4
Carnation Instant Breakfast	1 packet	80.0
Cheddar cheese	1 ounce	7.9
Cheerios cereal	1 cup	24.7
Chocolate-covered graham crackers	2	50.5
Chocolate skim milk	1 cup	45.5
Cocoa, sugar free with water	1 cup	42.5
Cod, baked/broiled	3 ounces	35.7
Corn, cooked	½ cup	26.2
Cottage cheese, 1%	1 cup	12.1
Cracker, rye	4 each	93.3
Cracklin Oat Bran cereal	1 cup	232.0
English Walnuts	¼ cup	47.4
Flaxseed	¼ cup	128.4
Grapefruit juice	1 cup	29.6
Green peas	1 cup	47.9
Hazelnuts, dried	¼ cup	46.9
Irish Steel-Cut Oats	½ cup dry or 1 cup cooked	215.9
Kasha, cooked	1 cup	437.5
Lima beans	1 cup	96.5
Long-grain brown rice, cooked	¾ cup	66.1
Low-fat granola	1 cup	89.9
Macadamia nuts	¼ cup	43.6

(continued)

Food	Amount	Milligrams
Millet, cooked	⅞ cup	57.0
Molasses	1 tablespoon	49.6
Mushrooms, shiitake, dried	5 each	24.8
Navy beans, cooked	1 cup	107.3
Oat bran, dry	¼ cup	55.2
Oatmeal, instant	1 packet	42.0
Old-fashioned oats	½ cup dry or 1 cup cooked	107.9
Orange juice	1 cup	27.3
Peanut granola bar	1 each	26.0
Peanuts, dry roasted	¼ cup	64.2
Pecans	¼ cup	34.6
Pine nuts, dried	¼ cup	79.2
Popcorn, air popped	3 cups	31.4
Pumpkin seeds, roasted	¼ cup	41.9
Quinoa, cooked	⅝ cup	89.3
Raisins	¼ cup	13.6
Red kidney beans, cooked	1 cup	85.0
Rye, whole grain (uncooked)	¼ cup	51.1
Salmon, baked/broiled	3 ounces	30.0
Skim milk	1 cup	39.5
Skim milk powder	¼ cup	91.9
Smooth peanut butter	2 tablespoons	50.2
Soy nuts, roasted	¼ cup	62.4
Spaghetti noodles, spinach, dry	1 ounce (about 1 cup cooked)	49.3
Split peas, cooked	½ cup	35.3
Sun-dried tomatoes	1 cup	104.7
Tahini (sesame butter)	1 tablespoon	53.0
Textured Vegetable Protein (TVP)	2 ounces	177.4

(continued)

Food	Amount	Milligrams
Tofu, silken, firm	½ cup	33.7
Total Wheat cereal	1 cup	42.8
Vanilla/fruit frozen yogurt	1 cup	32.1
Wheat germ, toasted	¼ cup	90.4
Wheaties cereal	1 cup	30.7
Whole wheat bagel, 100%	1	59.4
Whole wheat English muffin	1	38.5
Whole wheat flour	¼ cup	41.4
Wild rice, cooked	1 cup	70.8

Chromium

The interest in chromium as a mineral that may help people with diabetes also stems from the function it performs in the body. Chromium is intimately involved with energy metabolism. It helps regulate blood sugars; in fact, getting enough chromium may be especially important for people with diabetes. (Again, note the distinction between getting enough and taking a supplement to get extra.)

Like most nutrients, chromium plays other essential roles in the body, including:

- Helps the body use amino acids
- Assists the body in lipid, or fat, metabolism
- Aids in transmitting genetic information
- Involved in nerve-to-nerve message transmission
- Possibly reduces the effects of heart disease

Here are some important details about chromium: It is an essential component of a compound known as glucose tolerance factor (GTF). While its exact role is not defined, GTF appears to play a role in insulin-mediated glucose transport. Researchers have repeatedly found that people who are deficient in chromium tend to have more glucose intolerance than those who are not deficient. Ensuring adequate intake often helps normalize glucose metabolism and the body's response to insulin. Research also finds that correcting chromium deficiency improves lipid, or blood fat, abnormalities.

So the question is "Does taking extra chromium improve diabetic control?" The answer is that we do not know. The weight of the current evidence does not justify recommending chromium amounts over and above the recommended intake. As with much medical research, some studies have found a benefit while others have not. Until the research weighs clearly in favor of taking a supplement, the best advice is to make sure you are getting an adequate amount.

Beware of potentially dangerous and certainly untrue claims. Some supplement proponents make sensational claims about chromium and chromium picolinate. For example, you may have heard that chromium can melt away fat and/or convert fat to muscle. There simply is no research to justify this claim. While we may look for the magic bullet that will help us melt away unwanted pounds, the only thing that truly works is exercise and eating less. (Yes, I know this is a boring answer—but it's true!)

Here's a look at what you need and how to get it in real food:

Safe and Adequate Intake over Age 19
Men: 35 mcg per day
Women: 25 mcg per day

CHROMIUM

Food	Amount	Micrograms
Flaxseed	¼ cup	0.2
Wheat bran	¼ cup	0.5
Pickle	1	1.0
Barley	¼ cup dry or ¾ cup cooked	1.3
Barley, cooked	1 cup	2.5
Vegetable burger, frozen	1	3.7

(continued)

Food	Amount	Micrograms
Applesauce	1 cup	5.1
Textured vegetable protein, fortified	¼ cup	7.0
Broccoli	1 cup	7.6
Onion, green, raw	1/2 cup	7.8
Tomatoes, chopped	1 cup	9.0
Tomato	1	9.1
Cornmeal, yellow, whole grain	¼ cup	10.0
Cornmeal, white, whole grain	¼ cup	10.0
Oats, whole grain, uncooked	½ cup	11.0
Mushrooms, whole	8 each	13.0
Lettuce, Bibb	4 ounces	16.0
Lettuce, leaf	4 ounces	16.0
Lettuce, iceberg	4 ounces	16.0
Lettuce, romaine	4 ounces	16.0
Onion, yellow, cooked	½ cup	16.3
Onion, white, cooked	½ cup	16.3
Sauerkraut	1 cup	21.4
Turkey bologna	2 ounces	23.3
Balance Nutrition Bar (some flavors)	1	30.0
Cantaloupe	1 cup	37.0
Papaya	1	54.7

Zinc

Zinc plays a key role in both the formation and the action of insulin, not just in people with diabetes but in everyone. Diabetes researchers know that in people who are deficient in zinc, the pancreas (the islets of Langerhans in the pancreas, to be exact) may not be as efficient at producing and secreting insulin. We also know that some of the complications of having blood sugars running higher than normal cause the body to produce more intracellular oxidants and free radicals. In turn, these use up zinc at a greatly accelerated rate. This is because zinc is a co-factor, or ingredient, in many antioxidant enzymes. The bottom line is that people who do not take in enough zinc may suffer more of the cellular damage that underlies the classic complications of diabetes.

A study of women with Type 2 diabetes published in the *Journal of the American College of Nutrition* in 1998 found that these women were more likely to have moderate zinc deficiency and oxidant stress. They were also more likely to have low levels of zinc in their blood, and to have symptoms associated with zinc deficiency, such as decreased taste acuity.

Still, however, diabetes experts do not recommend zinc supplementation over and above requirements of the RDA.

Recommended Dietary Allowance over Age 19
Men: 11 mg per day
Women: 8 mg per day
My recommendation for men and women with diabetes: 15 mg per day

ZINC

Food	Amount	Milligrams
Baked potato with skin	1	0.4
Extra-firm light tofu	6 ounces	0.4
Macadamia nuts	¼ cup	0.4
Peanut granola bar	1	0.5
Salmon fillet, baked/broiled	3 ounces	0.5
Apricots, dried	½ cup	0.6
Coconut, toasted	1 ounce	0.6
Shrimp, steamed	2 (10 grams)	0.6
Bulgur wheat, cooked	⅝ cup	0.7
Hazelnuts	¼ cup	0.7
Oat bran, dry	¼ cup	0.7
Wheaties cereal	1 cup	0.7
Whole wheat pita pocket	1 each	0.7
Millet, dry	⅞ cup	0.8

(continued)

Food	Amount	Milligrams
Popcorn, air popped	3 cups	0.8
Spaghetti noodles, spinach, dry	1 ounce	0.8
Cheddar cheese	1 ounce	0.9
Chicken breast, skinless, roasted	3 ounces	0.9
Honey-Nut Cheerios cereal	1 cup	0.9
Long-grain brown rice, dry	¾ cup	0.9
Mozzarella cheese	1 ounce	0.9
Oatmeal, instant	1 packet	0.9
Peanut butter, chunky	2 tablespoons	0.9
Peanut butter, smooth	2 tablespoons	0.9
Salmon, canned	3 ounces	0.9
Walnuts	¼ cup	0.9
Whole wheat flour	¼ cup	0.9
Almonds, slivered	¼ cup	1.0
Scallops, baked	3 ounces	1.0
Split peas, cooked	½ cup	1.0
Swiss cheese	1 ounce	1.0
Brazil nuts	5	1.1
Sun-dried tomatoes	1 cup	1.1
Brewer's yeast	2 tablespoons	1.2
Buttermilk, dried	¼ cup	1.2
Low-fat cheddar cheese	1 ounce	1.2
Low-fat Colby cheese	1 ounce	1.2
Peanuts, dry roasted	¼ cup	1.2
Rolled oats, dry	½ cup	1.2
String cheese, mozzarella	1 ounce	1.2
Old-fashioned oats, dry	½ cup	1.3
Pecans	¼ cup	1.3
Sardines, oil packed	3.5 ounces	1.3
Swordfish, baked	3 ounces	1.3

(continued)

Food	Amount	Milligrams
Whole wheat bagel, 100%	1 each	1.3
Mushrooms, shiitake, dried	5	1.4
Quinoa, dry	⅝ cup	1.4
Soy nuts, roasted	¼ cup	1.4
Almonds, honey roasted	2 ounces	1.5
Nutri-Grain Strawberry Cereal Bar	1	1.5
Pine nuts, dried	¼ cup	1.5
Red kidney beans, cooked	1 cup	1.5
Amaranth	¼ cup	1.6
Rye, whole grain	¼ cup	1.6
Tahini (sesame butter)	1 tablespoon	1.6
Whole grain oats	¼ cup	1.6
Broad beans (fava beans), cooked	1 cup	1.7
Pumpkin seeds, roasted	¼ cup	1.7
Sunflower seeds, dry roasted	¼ cup	1.7
Pork chops, baked	3 ounces	1.8
Black beans, cooked	1 cup	1.9
Lima beans, cooked	1 cup	1.9
Navy beans, cooked	1 cup	1.9
Bran Flakes cereal	1 cup	2.0
Cranberry beans, boiled	1 cup	2.0
Soybeans, boiled	1 cup	2.0
White beans, cooked	1 cup	2.0
Multi-Grain Flakes cereal	1 cup	2.1
Rye crackers	4	2.2
Wild rice, cooked	1 cup	2.2
Skim milk powder	¼ cup	2.4
Lentils, cooked	1 cup	2.5
Flaxseed	¼ cup	2.6
Irish Steel-Cut Oats, dry	½ cup	2.6

(continued)

Food	Amount	Milligrams
Almond nuts, toasted	2 ounces	2.8
Cheerios cereal	1 cup	2.8
Ham	3 ounces	2.8
Fruit & Fiber cereal with dates, raisins, and nuts	1 cup	3.0
Instant breakfast	1 packet	3.0
Textured Vegetable Protein (TVP)	2 ounces	3.0
Turkey, dark meat	3 ounces	3.3
Crab, baked/broiled	3 ounces	3.4
Special K cereal	1 cup	3.8
Beef roast	3 ounces	4.0
Adzuki beans, cooked	1 cup	4.1
Raisin Bran cereal	1 cup	4.2
Wheat germ, toasted	¼ cup	4.7
Kasha, cooked	1 cup	4.8
Beef flank steak, cooked	3 ounces	4.9
Ground beef, extra lean	3.5 ounces	5.4
All-Bran cereal	1 cup	7.5
Kellogg's Lowfat Granola	1 cup	12.9
Total wheat cereal	1 cup	20.0
Oysters, baked/broiled	3 ounces	38.4

Vitamin E

Of all vitamins, E boasts the longest and most diverse list of potential benefits—from reducing the risk of heart disease and adult-onset diabetes to improving exercise performance. Expecting to gain at least some advantage, consumers will often take ten or even one hundred times the Recommended Dietary Allowance; others squeeze the glistening gel onto their skin, hoping to erase scars and wrinkles. But what is true and what is a snake-oil promise?

Vitamin E was named *tocopherol,* from the Greek *tos* for childbirth and *phero* meaning to bring forth, after scientists discovered in 1922 that it prevented fetal death in animals. Thirty to forty years later researchers found that humans literally cannot live without vitamin E. It is not one but several compounds, tocopherols and tocotrienols, that vary widely in their "active" vitamin E content. Alpha-tocopherol is both the most biologically active and the most widely distributed in nature.

Vitamin E deficiency is rare, occurring only in premature infants and people who do not absorb fat normally; adult deficiencies take five to ten years to develop. The Recommended Dietary Allowance (RDA) to prevent the signs of anemia, fragile red blood cells, and neurological abnormalities is 15 milligrams for men and women (equivalent to 22.5 IU). That is in sharp contrast to amounts proposed for vitamin E's other touted benefits—100 to 800 IU.

Why the colossal discrepancy? As we probe the relationship between vitamin E and disease, we have to start somewhere and basically guess at potentially helpful doses. In contrast, assigning recommended allowances for essential nutrients is relatively easy and more exacting: We search for the dose that prevents deficiencies (adding a generous pinch of safety). Researchers withdrew vitamin C, for example, until gums started to bleed (a symptom of deficiency) and then added it back until bleeding disappeared.

But quantifying a nutrient's role in disease prevention is more challenging, and here researchers are in unfamiliar territory. The line marking the start of a chronic disease process isn't as sharp as the one defining the beginning of an acute nutrient deficiency. For example, if a nutrient purportedly guards against cancer, we cannot measure exactly how much of the nutrient arrests cancer because we don't fully understand cancer's genesis.

New studies on vitamin E have shown that food intakes of just tens of units seem to confer the same benefit as hundreds of supplemental units. But we must note that when studies correlate vitamin E benefits with higher food intake, the vitamin E might simply be a marker for a healthier diet that *as a whole* confers the benefits. People who get vitamin E from food, for example, generally consume diets packed with other disease-fighting substances, such as fiber, folic acid, and phytonutrients. That is not to say that vitamin E isn't important, just that it may take less vitamin E if several protective factors work together. Getting enough vitamin C, for example, may recycle vitamin E or help the body use it again and again.

Old job, new roles.   The new roles for vitamin E focus on its job as the body's key chain-breaking antioxidant, or scavenger of cell-damaging free radicals. By neutralizing these stray high-energy particles that otherwise ricochet wildly, scarring and punching holes in cells, vitamin E could theoretically prevent many chronic diseases. Now research is beginning to bridge the theoretical and the possible.

"Despite many claims and promising data, vitamin E has not been *proven* to prevent any disease," notes vitamin E maven Herbert J. Kayden, M.D., professor of medicine at New York University Medical Center. "We simply don't have the type of cause-and-effect proof that we have, for example, with penicillin and its ability to cure pneumococcus."

Heart disease.   Vitamin E's role in protecting against heart disease is at best confusing. For many years heart disease researchers found consistently that people who took 200 to 400 IU of vitamin E had less risk of coronary artery disease. This interest in vitamin E started in the late 1980s when researchers reported that LDL ("bad") cholesterol particles damaged by free radicals (referred to as oxidized) were more likely to clog the heart's arteries. Subsequent test tube research found that adding vitamin E to LDL cholesterol rendered the bad cholesterol oxidation resistant. Vitamin E may confer additional protection against heart diseast: In test tubes it stops excessive muscle cell formation in damaged arteries and keeps blood clotting in check. Both of these processes ultimately clog arteries.

Population-based studies of vitamin E intake and heart disease risk have had mixed results. While three American studies and a Finnish study found that both men and women with higher vitamin E intakes had lower coronary disease risk—by at least one-third and possibly by as much as two-thirds—other studies have had negative results. The vitamin E dose associated with this decreased risk varies widely, from just 10 IU daily obtained from food to an average of about 200 IU in supplemental form.

The HOPE (Heart Outcomes Prevention Evaluation) study, published in the January 20, 2000, issue of the *New England Journal of Medicine,* found that a highly significant cardiovascular protection was provided by an angiotensin-converting enzyme inhibitor, ramipril, at a dose of 10 milligrams per day, after a follow-up of four and a half years. However, the study did not find a benefit of vitamin E supplements at a dose of 400 IU per day in high-risk patients (over 55 years old) who had evidence of vascular disease (secondary prevention) or combined diabetes and another cardiovascular risk factor (primary prevention).

So what should you do about this supplement? My advice is to make sure you get as much as possible through your diet. It is difficult to get enough through diet because many sources of vitamin E are very high in fat (vitamin E is a fat-soluble vitamin and therefore tends to travel with fattier foods). See the chart below for some excellent low-fat sources of vitamin E. Included in the chart are other nutrients found in quantity in the foods. As you can see, choosing foods high in vitamin E is an automatic home run in terms of getting additional nutrients. One other note: If you take a multivitamin, you'll make up the difference between what is needed for good health and higher levels (that you cannot get through diet), which may reduce heart disease risk.

Foods Rich in Vitamin E

It is possible to get at least 10 IU of vitamin E without eating a lot of high-fat foods. Use this chart to boost your intake of vitamin E and yet follow a diet that meets the American Heart Association's guidelines for limiting fat, especially saturated fat. You will also be acquiring many other key nutrients that may help fight heart disease and cancer, and keep you healthy in general.

Food	Serving Size	IU per Serving	Bonus Nutrients
Asparagus, steamed	1 cup	2.7	Fiber, vitamin C, folate, iron, potassium
Beet greens, boiled	1 cup	3.0	Fiber, beta-carotene, vitamin C, calcium, iron, potassium
Broccoli, boiled	1 cup	2.6	Fiber, vitamin C, folate, calcium, iron, potassium
Cabbage, raw, shredded	1 cup	1.7	Fiber, vitamin C

(continued)

Food	Serving Size	IU per Serving	Bonus Nutrients
Cabbage, boiled	1 cup	3.7	Fiber, vitamin C
Dandelion greens, boiled	1 cup	3.1	Fiber, beta-carotene, calcium, iron, potassium, vitamin C
Mustard greens, boiled	1 cup	4.2	Fiber, beta-carotene, vitamin C, folate, calcium, iron, potassium
Soybeans, boiled	1 cup	5.0	Fiber, calcium, iron, folate, potassium
Spinach, boiled	1 cup	3.5	Beta-carotene, folate, calcium, iron, potassium, vitamin C
Spinach, raw	1 cup	1.5	Beta-carotene, folate, calcium, iron, potassium, vitamin C
Sweet potato	1	0.7	Fiber, beta-carotene, vitamin C, potassium
Swiss chard, cooked	1 cup	1.8	Fiber, beta-carotene, vitamin C, calcium, iron, potassium
Tomato paste, canned	¼ cup	1.6	Vitamin C, iron, potassium
Tomato, raw	1 medium	1.5	Vitamin C, beta-carotene, potassium
Turnip green, boiled	1 cup	3.7	Fiber, beta-carotene, vitamin C, folate, calcium, iron, potassium
Yam, white, boiled	1 cup	9.2	Fiber, vitamin C, potassium
Almonds, whole, toasted	1 ounce	10.2	Fiber, calcium, iron
Filberts, dry or oil roasted	1 ounce	10.6	Fiber, calcium, iron
Peanut butter	2 tablespoons	3.6	Iron, folate, protein, fiber

(continued)

202

Food	Serving Size	IU per Serving	Bonus Nutrients
Peanuts	1 ounce	3.1	Iron, folate, protein, fiber
Sunflower seeds	1 tablespoon	6.7	Iron
Blueberries	1 cup	2.2	Fiber, vitamin C, potassium
Guava	1	1.5	Fiber, vitamin C, potassium
Kiwifruit	1	1.3	Vitamin C, fiber, potassium
Papaya	1	5.1	Vitamin C, fiber, potassium
Prunes	10	1.7	Fiber, vitamin C, potassium
Barley	1 cup	1.8	B vitamins, minerals, fiber
Quinoa, uncooked	½ cup	6.2	B vitamins, minerals, fiber
Wheat germ, toasted	2 tablespoons	4.2	B vitamins, minerals, fiber
Catfish, steamed	3 ounces	1.9	
Crab, baked/broiled	3 ounces	2.1	
Halibut, baked/broiled	3 ounces	0.9	
Salmon, steamed	3 ounces	2.4	Omega-3 fatty acids
Shrimp, steamed	3 ounces	2.2	
Sole, poached	3 ounces	3.0	
Tuna steak, baked/broiled	3 ounces	2.5	
Chicken breast, skinless, baked	3 ounces	0.2	
Chicken thigh, skinless, baked	3 ounces	0.6	
Turkey meat, dark, baked	3 ounces	0.8	
Canola oil	1 tablespoon	4.7	
Corn oil	1 tablespoon	4.3	
Olive oil	1 tablespoon	2.4	
Sunflower oil	1 tablespoon	12.2	

Should I Take a Vitamin/Mineral Supplement?

People in all walks of life and in every type of health situation ask this question, wondering if they should take a supplement "just to be on the safe side."

If you eat the types of meals outlined in this book, then most likely you do not need a supplement. The possible exceptions to this rule are as follows:

- Chromium, magnesium, and zinc: Most people come up just slightly short on these minerals when they depend on diet alone. That is why it is recommended that you choose a vitamin/mineral supplement which supplies about 100 percent of the recommended intake for all nutrients.

But don't go overboard and take more than that. Also, I do not recommend single supplements—one pill of zinc, one pill of chromium, one of magnesium, etc. The best possible situation is to take one supplement that supplies all of these. An excellent example is Centrum—From A to Zinc. Research has also found that Centrum is consistently one of the best-absorbed nutrient supplements.

- If you have a special condition that prevents you from getting all nutrients, such as a gastrointestinal problem with absorbing nutrients, then you may need to supplement certain ones. Your health care provider will know for sure.
- People who cannot have dairy products or do not eat enough of them may also need to supplement calcium and possibly vitamin D. The multivitamin supplement will supply vitamin D and a small amount of calcium. If you are not getting 1,000 to 1,500 milligrams of calcium daily, then be sure to take a calcium supplement. If you take a multivitamin/mineral supplement, choose a calcium supplement *without* vitamin D, or you will get too much D.
  - —Calcium citrate and calcium carbonate are the best-absorbed types of calcium supplements.

—Take your supplement at the correct time. (See the sidebar about timing supplements.)

—Avoid so-called natural supplements; calcium supplements made from bone meal, oyster shells, and dolomite may contain lead.

- Menstruating women may need iron, especially if they do not acquire enough through their diet.

- Vegans and some vegetarians—and others who do not eat foods of animal origin—need to pay special attention to getting enough vitamin B_{12}.

- After age 60, nutrient needs may change. For example, the body loses its ability to synthesize vitamin D and to absorb vitamin B_{12}. Your health care provider will know when and if you might need to begin supplementing these nutrients after age 60.

Do's and Don'ts for Taking Supplements

Here are some quick tips on supplements:

- Take your multivitamin with a meal. A full stomach takes longer to empty, and this extra time gives the multivitamin more time to break down and dissolve—which means you get more of it.

- If you take a calcium supplement, take calcium carbonate with meals and take calcium citrate either between or with meals. If you take 1,000 milligrams of a calcium supplement, take it in divided doses because then the body will absorb more of it.

- If you take a calcium supplement and an iron supplement (or a multivitamin containing iron), take them at separate times. Calcium and iron compete for absorption.

- Don't buy chelated vitamins. There is no evidence that they offer benefits. Instead buy some fresh asparagus or a papaya.

- Don't buy time-released supplements. There is no evidence of their benefits, and it would be better to buy fresh watercress and fresh raspberries with the money you save.

- If you eat less than 1,500 calories in an attempt to lose weight, you might not be able to get all your nutrients in your diet. Reach for a multivitamin/mineral supplement that supplies no more than 100 percent of the recommended intake.

- During recovery from a serious illness, surgery, or injury, the body may need extra nutrients, and taking one multivitamin may help. If you take cortisone medications, ask your physician about taking extra vitamin A. *This should only be done with a doctor's advice because taking too much vitamin A can quickly lead to vitamin A toxicity.*

- If you take certain medications, you may need to pay attention to getting certain nutrients (see table on pages 208 and 209).

- Taking vitamin E (see pages 198–201).

Herbs and Other Supplements

Today, the number of herbs on the market is daunting. Even more daunting is the huge number of claims for each of these herbs. First I'll discuss a few of the herbs that have gotten some attention in the diabetes arena. Then I'm going to summarize the best available evidence (by no means complete, though) about herbs with potential dangers.

Herbal Terminology

Let's begin with a few herb terminology basics. Herbs are found in various forms and formulations. Some of the terms you will see include the following:

Infusion: A tea brewed in a teapot with loose tea leaves and then strained.

Decoction: A gentle simmering process used to extract the medicinal substance of fibrous plant material.

Tincture: A highly concentrated alcohol-based liquid herbal extract.

Herbal bath: A fifteen- to thirty-minute soak in warm water with herbs, herbal tea, or essential oil.

Compress: A cloth soaked in a hot or cold herbal preparation (infusion, decoction, or diluted tincture) to relieve muscle or joint aches, wounds, or cramps.

Poultice: An herbal wrap consisting of a dampened mixture of chopped or bruised herbs held in place on the skin by a wet piece of gauze.

Liniment: A concentrated herbal extract used externally to treat skin problems or muscle aches.

Infused oil: A vegetable oil base infused with herbs.

Syrups and lozenges: Concentrated decoctions or infusions of herbs mixed with honey or sugar.

Cream: An emulsion of oil- and water-based ingredients.

Suppository: A medicated compound designed to be slipped into the rectum or vagina.

Salves and ointments: Medicated substances that form a protective and soothing layer on the skin.

Herbs and Other Supplements Making News in Diabetes Literature

Research has called attention to a couple of herbs and their potential to help people with diabetes. Please note that this research is in no way final.

American ginseng. Some research suggests that American ginseng may play a role in carbohydrate metabolism and therefore in diabetes. One study published in the *Archives of Internal Medicine* on April 10, 2000, reported on the effects of taking ginseng before or with 25 grams of glucose in both diabetics and nondiabetics. The researchers found a significant improvement in post-meal blood sugar levels when people with Type 2 diabetes took ginseng either forty minutes before or with 25 grams of glucose compared to a placebo. They also found that in people without diabetes, the ginseng caused somewhat of a drop in postprandial blood sugars, compared to a placebo. While this study does indeed hint at some promising results, it

NUTRIENT–DRUG INTERACTIONS

Drug Group	Generic Name	Sample Brand Names	Nutrients Possibly Affected
Antacids	Sodium bicarbonate Aluminum hydroxide	Alka-Seltzer Amphojel, Basaljel, Maalox	Folic acid, phosphate, calcium, copper
Antibacterial agents	Boric acid Trimethoprim Isoniazid	— Bactrim, Sulfatrim Nydrazid, Rifamate	Vitamins B_2, B_6, and D, folic acid, niacin
Antibiotics	Tetracycline Gentamicin Cephalosporins	Achromycin Garamycin Cefamandole	Iron, calcium, potassium, magnesium, vitamin K
Anticancer drugs	Methotrexate Cisplatin	Methotrexate Platinol	Folic acid, calcium, magnesium
Anticonvulsants	Phenytoin Phenobarbital Primidone Valproic acid	Dilantin Donnatal Mysoline Depakene	Folic acid, vitamins D and K
Anticoagulants	Warfarin	Coumadin	Vitamin K
Anti-inflammatory agents	Aspirin Indomethacin Methotrexate Penicillamine Prednisone Sulfasalazine	Bayer, Bufferin, Ecotrin Indocin Rheumatrex Cuprimine, Depen Deltasone, Sterapred Azulfidine	Vitamin C, folic acid, iron, calcium, zinc, copper, vitamin B_6, potassium

Drug Group	Generic Name	Sample Brand Names	Nutrients Possibly Affected
Antimalarials	Pyrimethamine	Daraprim, Fansidar	Folic acid
Cholesterol-lowering medications	Cholestryamine Colestipol	Questran Colestid	Vitamins A, D, E, K, B_{12}, and folic acid
Diuretics	Thiazides Furosemide Ethacrynic acid Hydralazine Triamterene	Diucardin, Diuril Lasix Edecrin Apresazide, Apresoline Dyrenium	Potassium, magnesium, calcium, vitamin B_6, folic acid
Laxatives	Mineral oil Pheolphthalein Senna	Fleet Agoral, Alophen Dosaflex, Senokot	Vitamins A, D, and K, potassium, calcium
Contraceptives	Oral contraceptives	Modicon, Nordette, Ortho-Novum, Triphasil	Vitamins B_6 and C, folic acid
Tranquilizers	Chlorpromazine	Thorazine	Vitamin B_2

is too early to comment on the long-term efficacy of using ginseng. More studies are needed, such as one that would study HbA1c (glycosylated hemoglobin, an index of average blood glucose levels over three months) over a longer period of time.

Alfalfa.   You may have read that taking a supplement of alfalfa mixed with other herbal constituents will lower blood sugar levels. These studies, however, have primarily been conducted in mice; human studies are lacking. There is insufficient evidence to recommend taking alfalfa-based supplements to lower blood sugar.

Aloe vera.   A very limited number of animal and human experimental studies have been done in which subjects who were given the dried sap of the aloe vera plant experienced a slight reduction in blood sugar levels. But there is inadequate evidence at this time to recommend that people with diabetes eat aloe vera sap.

Fish oil supplements.   This is a difficult subject to discuss. To be sure, eating fish is thought to be a tremendous help in battling heart disease, which is especially important for people with diabetes. But what about fish oil supplements? Fish and heart disease experts say that fish oil supplements are at best controversial. In fact, taking fish oil supplements may even backfire on people with diabetes. Here's why: Fish oil supplements have quite a few calories; after all, they are entirely fat. If you eat regular meals and get all your recommended calories from food, and then take fish oil supplements, on top of that, you most likely would get too many calories. The effect of too many calories is obvious: You could gain weight, or you might not lose the weight you need to.

What about eating fish? As discussed earlier, including at least two and as many as four fish meals weekly is a great idea.

Herbs That May Be Dangerous

Some herbs may cause serious health problems and/or can interact with medications to produce dangerous side effects. In addition to those noted here, be aware that certain people have individual sensitivities and allergies to other herbs. To be safe, always check with your physician before taking an herb, especially if you have known allergies.

Herbs to Avoid

The following herbs are toxic and should never be used by anyone because the risks far outweigh the benefits:

Aconite: Has resulted in numerous poisonings in China.

Belladonna: Contains three toxic alkaloids, including atropine.

Blue cohosh: Can induce abortion.

Borage: May contain liver toxins and carcinogens.

Broom: May slow heart rhythm; contains toxic alkaloids.

Burdock: Can cause atropine poisoning if adulterated with root of belladonna or deadly nightshade.

Chaparral: Can cause severe hepatitis and liver failure.

Comfrey: Contains toxins linked to liver disease and death.

Ephedra (ma huang): Contains cardiac toxins that elevate blood pressure and cause palpitations and stroke; has been linked to dozens of deaths.

Germander: Contains a stimulant that can cause heart problems.

Jin bu huan: Used as a sedative; in some children has caused liver toxicity and severe breathing problems.

Kombucha tea: Can cause liver damage and intestinal problems.

Lobelia: Large doses can cause rapid heartbeat, coma, and death.

Pennyroyal: Can cause liver damage, convulsions, abortions, coma, and death.

Poke root: Extremely toxic; can result in low blood pressure and respiratory depression.

Sassafras: Contains the carcinogen *safrole*. Banned from use in food.

Skullcap: Can cause liver damage.

Sleeping Buddha: May cause excessive sedation in all users; may cause fetal damage when used by pregnant women.

Stephania and **magnolia:** Renal toxic (used as a weight-loss product in Belgium, it has resulted in kidney transplantation in twenty patients).

Tryptophan: May cause eosinophilia-myalgia syndrome.

Wormwood: Can cause convulsions, loss of consciousness, and hallucinations.

Yohimbe: May have monoamine oxidase inhibitory activity and may interact with antidepressants. Can cause weakness, paralysis, gastrointestinal problems, psychosis, paralysis, and death. Risk-to-benefit ratio is too high to recommend its use.

Herbs to Use with Caution

The following herbs may cause problems in people with certain conditions who are taking particular medications or who are especially sensitive:

Chamomile: Should be avoided by people with ragweed allergy; can cause severe allergic reaction.

Echinacea: Should not be taken by people with autoimmune diseases such as multiple sclerosis and systemic lupus erythematosus or by people who are HIV-positive. Long-term use by anyone may suppress the immune system rather than help it. Most herbal experts advise taking echinacea for a couple of months and then stopping for a month.

Feverfew: May interfere with blood clotting; should be discontinued before surgery.

Ginger: May interfere with blood clotting; should be discontinued before surgery.

Ginkgo: Increases chance of excess bleeding in people taking anticoagulant and antiplatelet drugs. Not safe for children.

Goldenseal: Interferes with short-acting anticoagulant medications.

Hawthorn: Should not be taken by people on heart medications. May interfere with digoxin monitoring.

Kava-Kava: May increase suicidal tendency in people with endogenous depression. Not safe for pregnant and nursing women or people with Parkinson's disease.

Licorice: May cause excessive potassium loss in people taking potassium-losing medications.

St. John's Wort: May enhance effects of narcotics, SSRIs (selective serotonin reuptake inhibitors), and alcohol. May cause photosensitivity, especially in fair-skinned people. High doses may cause peripheral neuropathy.

Valerian: Enhances effect of sedatives. May cause morning drowsiness and difficulty walking. Cases of severe liver damage have been reported. May have excitatory effect in some people.

Herbs with Potential Cardiac Drug Interactions

Because so many people with diabetes are at risk for heart disease, presented here are herbs that when interacting with cardiac medications can have potentially undesirable results.

Barberry: Counteracts short-acting anticoagulants.

Bromelain (from pineapple): May increase bleeding risk when taken with anticoagulants.

Garlic: May enhance the action of anticoagulant and antiplatelet drugs (which may lead to excessive bleeding).

Ginkgo: Enhances the action of anticoagulant and antiplatelet drugs.

Goldenseal: Counteracts short-acting anticoagulants.

Grapefruit juice: Dangerous when combined with calcium channel blockers.

Hawthorn: May enhance actions of cardiac glycosides, which can be dangerous.

Licorice: May worsen effect of drugs that cause potassium loss.

Oregon grape: Counteracts short-acting anticoagulants.

Stimulant laxatives: These include senna leaf and fruit, cascara sagrada bark, aloe vera leaf (not gel), buckthorn bark and berry, and rhubarb. May cause potassium loss, which may strengthen the effects of cardiac glycosides and antiarrhythmic agents. Simultaneous use of thiazide diuretics, corticosteroids, or licorice root increases potassium loss.

Chapter Eleven

Products That Help

What products on the grocery store shelf can help you, as a diabetic, eat more healthfully and control your blood sugar? You will be happy to learn that the legwork and label reading has been done for you. As you might expect, products and brands change over time, so you will also find here some guidelines of what to look for in certain products.

Cold Cereals

Look for a cold cereal that has no more than 2 to 3 grams of fat per serving and also at least 2 grams, and preferably 3 or 4, of fiber per serving. The saturated fat content should be zero. Finally, if you're going with a cold cereal, this is one great way of getting oats, an excellent source of soluble fiber.

Name	Brand	Serving Size	Calories	Fat	Saturated Fat	Cholesterol	Sodium	Total Carbohydrates	Dietary Fiber	Protein
Complete Oat Bran Flakes	Kellogg's	¾ cup	110	1.0	0	0	210	23	4	3
Harmony	General Mills	1¼ cups	200	1.0	0	0	350	44	2	5
Organic Oat Bran Flakes with Raisins	Health Valley	¾ cup	110	0	0	0	90	26	4	3
Smart Start	Kellogg's	1 cup	180	0.5	0	0	330	43	2	3
Cheerios	General Mills	1 cup	110	2.0	0	0	280	22	3	3

Hot Cereals

As with the cold cereals, the hot ones chosen are oat-based to obtain that wonderful soluble fiber. Note that the serving size (if not instant) is by the uncooked portion. Saturated fat should be less than 1 gram and fiber should be at least 4 grams per serving.

Name	Brand	Serving Size	Calories	Fat	Saturated Fat	Cholesterol	Sodium	Total Carbohydrates	Dietary Fiber	Protein
Oat Bran Hot Cereal	Old Wessex	⅓ cup	140	4.0	0.5	0	0	23	7	8.0
Instant Oatmeal	Quaker	1 packet	172	2.1	0.4	0	242	35.7	2.8	4.1
Old Fashioned Oatmeal	Quaker	½ cup	150	3.0	0.5	0	0	27	4	5.0

Dried Fruits

These fruits are a wonderful way to get fiber and potassium, both substances your body is looking for to fight diabetes and heart disease. You can't go wrong with dried fruits, and the ones listed here are highest in fiber. Avoid dried fruits that have sugar or corn syrup in the ingredient list.

Name	Brand	Serving Size	Calories	Fat	Saturated Fat	Cholesterol	Sodium	Total Carbohydrates	Dietary Fiber	Protein
Apricot	Fruitlings	⅓ cup	110	0	0	0	30	29	3	0
Chopped Dates	Dole	¼ cup	120	0	0	0	10	33	3	0
Pitted Dates	Dole	5–6	120	0	0	0	0	31	3	0
California Calimyrna Figs	Sun Maid	¼ cup (about 3 figs)	120	0	0	0	0	28	5	0
Mission Figlets	Orchard Choice	1½ ounces (about 5 figs)	120	0		0	0	28	5	0

Jellies/Jams

Breakfast toast without jam is certainly boring, so I've looked long and hard for the brands and types that contribute few calories and few carbohydrate grams. Some general guidelines to help you: Look for those that have 10 to 25 calories per tablespoon; obviously, choosing those at the lower end is better.

Name	Brand	Serving Size	Calories	Fat	Sodium
Low Sugar Red Raspberry	Smucker's	1 tablespoon	25	0	0
Light Boysenberry Preserves	Knott's Berry Farms	1 tablespoon	20	0	0
Light Sugar-Free Red Raspberry Preserves	Smucker's	1 tablespoon	10	0	0

Cheese

Cheese is a tough subject; take it from someone who could eat cheese for breakfast, lunch, and dinner! My first choice in cheese, in terms of health, should be soy cheeses. The best brand is Veggie Slices by Galaxy Foods. After that you can try the fat-free versions of dairy-based cheeses, but they are not great for melting. Some good light choices are also noted here.

Name	Brand	Serving Size	Calories	Fat	Saturated Fat	Cholesterol	Sodium	Total Carbohydrates	Dietary Fiber	Protein
Veggie Slices, American Flavor	Galaxy Foods	1 slice	40	2.0	0	0	260	1	0	4
Veggie Slices, Mozzarella Flavor	Galaxy Foods	1 slice	40	2.0	0	0	150	1	0	4
Fat-Free Mozzarella Singles	Kraft	1 slice	30	0	0	< 5	270	2	0	5
Fat-Free Swiss Singles	Borden	1 slice	30	0	0	0	310	2	0	5
Fat-Free Sharp Singles	Borden	1 slice	30	0	0	< 5	320	2	0	5
Light Shredded Mild Cheddar, Reduced Fat	Sargento	¼ cup	70	4.5	3	10	200	1	0	8
50% Less Fat, Jalapeño Cheddar Cheese	Cabot	1 ounce (1-inch cube)	70	4.5	3	15	170	1	0	8

(continued)

Cheese *(cont.)*

Name	Brand	Serving Size	Calories	Fat	Saturated Fat	Cholesterol	Sodium	Total Carbohydrates	Dietary Fiber	Protein
50% Less Fat, Vermont Cheddar Cheese	Cabot	1 ounce (1-inch cube)	70	4.5	3	15	170	1	0	8
100% Grated Parmesan Cheese	Kraft	2 tsp	20	1.5	1	<5	85	0	0	2
Veggie Topping, Parmesan Flavor	Galaxy Foods	2 tsp	15	0.5	0	0	80	0.5	0	2

Croutons

What is a great salad without croutons? Unfortunately, regular croutons are a virtual landmine of fat, but here are some wonderful fat-free versions you can enjoy.

Name	Brand	Serving Size	Calories	Fat	Saturated Fat	Cholesterol	Sodium	Total Carbohydrates	Dietary Fiber	Protein
Fat-Free Seasoned	Rothbury Farm	2 tbsp	25	0	0	0	105	5	0	0
Fat-Free Spicy Italian	Pepperidge Farm	6	30	0	0	0	90	5	0	0
Fat-Free Onion & Garlic	Pepperidge Farm	6	30	0	0	0	95	5	0	0
Fat-Free Caesar	Pepperidge Farm	6	30	0	0	0	80	5	0	0

Beans

While you've learned all about cooking your own beans (from dry) and freezing them, there are times when you just don't have that kind of time. Here are some wonderful canned versions. Note the sodium column; this is the amount for the portion unrinsed. If you place the beans in a strainer and rinse well with cold water, you can reduce this sodium by half (approximately).

Name	Brand	Serving Size	Calories	Fat	Saturated Fat	Cholesterol	Sodium	Total Carbohydrates	Dietary Fiber	Protein
Canned Pinto Beans	Bush's Best	½ cup	110	0.5	0	0	430	18	6	6
Canned Cannellini Beans (white kidney)	Progresso	½ cup	100	0.5	0	0	270	18	5	5
Organic Refried Beans, Black Beans w/Roasted Jalapeño	ShariAnn's	½ cup	110	0	0	0	390	20	4	8
Canned Dark Red Kidney Beans	Joan of Arc	½ cup	110	0	0	0	340	20	6	8
Canned Chickpeas	Hanover	½ cup	110	1	0	0	400	20	7	7
Canned Organic Black Beans	ShariAnn's	½ cup	90	0	0	0	100	16	4	6

Butter/Margarine

This is another confusing section in the grocery store. Even 100% canola-based margarines can contain trans fats that clog the arteries. The best advice is to choose a brand that says "Trans fat free" or "Contains no trans fatty acids" or something along those lines. There is only one such brand in my area.

Name	Brand	Serving Size	Calories	Fat	Saturated Fat	Cholesterol	Sodium	Total Carbohydrates	Dietary Fiber	Protein
Non-hydrogenated (no trans fatty acids)	Smart Balance	1 tbsp	80	9	2.5	0	90	0	0	0

Crackers

Here you want to watch the sodium and the fat in most cases, although in the best of all worlds you would want to find a cracker that is also high in fiber.

Name	Brand	Serving Size	Calories	Fat	Saturated Fat	Cholesterol	Sodium	Total Carbohydrates	Dietary Fiber	Protein
Ritz Crackers	Nabisco	5	80	4	1	0	135	10	0	1
Wheat Crackers	SnackRite	7	140	5	1	0	170	21	4	3
Reduced-fat Wheat Thins	Nabisco	16	130	4	1	0	260	21	1	2
Original Sesame Biscuits Crackers	Mariner Biscuit	5	60	1	0	0	115	10	0	2

Vegetable Alternatives for Meat

You can use this list of products in place of meat, such as for ground beef, Canadian bacon, pepperoni, and chicken. The huge advantage is that they have virtually no saturated fat and do have fiber; their total fat content is also much lower than the product they simulate. You owe it to yourself to try many of them!

Name	Brand	Serving Size	Calories	Fat	Saturated Fat	Cholesterol	Sodium	Total Carbohydrates	Dietary Fiber	Protein
Ground Meatless	MorningStar Farms	½ cup	60	0	0	0	260	4.0	2.0	10.0
Canadian Veggie Bacon	Yves	3 slices	80	0.5	0	0	480	1.0	1.0	17.0
Veggie Pizza Pepperoni	Yves	16 slices	70	0	0	0	480	4.0	3.0	14.0
Meatless Nuggets	Boca	4 nuggets	189	6.96	1.8	1.7	567	15.7	2.4	15.9
Spicy Chik'N Patties	Boca	1 patty	151	6.11	0.5	2.1	469	11.5	2.0	12.6
Smoked Sausages	Boca	1 link	125	5.47	0.6	0	895	6.6	1.7	12.4
Roasted Onion Burger	Boca	1 patty	94	1.28	0.1	0.7	463	7.9	5.0	12.8
Chef Max's Favorite Burger	Boca	1 patty	110	3.48	0.9	4.5	373	5.6	3.6	14.1
Original Chik'N Patties	Boca	1 patty	151	6.11	0.5	2.1	469	11.5	2.0	12.6
Bratwurst Sausages	Boca	1 link	129	6.53	0.7	0.6	872	5.7	1.1	12.0

(continued)

Vegetable Alternatives *(cont.)*

Name	Brand	Serving Size	Calories	Fat	Saturated Fat	Cholesterol	Sodium	Total Carbohydrates	Dietary Fiber	Protein
Italian Sausages	Boca	1 link	135	6.74	0.6	0	1,006	7.5	2.6	11.0
Grilled Vegetable Burger	Boca	1 patty	84	0.92	0.5	0.1	305	5.8	4.6	13.1
Roasted Garlic Naturally Flavored Burger	Boca	1 patty	101	2.06	0.7	2.5	395	6.5	5.3	14.2
Salsa Burger	Boca	1 patty	92	0.78	0.4	2.3	379	8.0	5.2	13.4
Original Vegan Burger	Boca	1 patty	89	1.21	0.2	0	350	6.0	3.9	13.4
Meatless Crumbles	Boca	1 cup	79	0.74	0.1	0	293	6.4	1.0	12.1
Breakfast Links	Boca	1 link	98	4.05	0.4	0	328	5.9	3.7	9.6
Breakfast Patties	Boca	1 patty	85	3.76	0.3	0	261	4.6	3.0	8.0

Ready-to-Eat Fish (Canned)

As you've learned in this book, you simply cannot get enough fish in your diet. It is not always possible to buy fresh, so please try the canned ones. Just choose them canned in water and drain the liquid; this reduces the sodium by about half.

Name	Brand	Serving Size	Calories	Fat	Saturated Fat	Cholesterol	Sodium	Total Carbohydrates	Dietary Fiber	Protein
Chunk Light Tuna in Spring Water	Star Kist	2 ounces	60	0.5	0	30	250	0	0	13
Solid White Albacore Tuna in Spring Water	Star Kist	2 ounces	73	1.6	0	23	213	0	0	13
Canned Red Salmon	Pillar Rock	¼ cup	110	7.0	1.5	0	270	0	0	13
Anchovies, jar	Bellino	6 pieces	25	1.5	0	0	750	0	0	4

Pasta

If you can put some color in your pasta, you will increase the fiber (white pasta doesn't have fiber). As you've learned, fiber helps slow the absorption of foods, which slows the rise in blood sugar.

Name	Brand	Serving Size	Calories	Fat	Saturated Fat	Cholesterol	Sodium	Total Carbohydrates	Dietary Fiber	Protein
Whole Wheat Whole Grain Lasagna Noodles	Hodgson Mill	2 ounces, uncooked	190	1	0	0	10	34	6	9
Enriched Spinach Egg Noodles	Mrs. Weiss	2 ounces, uncooked (about 1 cup)	210	2	0.5	50	20	40	2	8
Tri-color Rotini Pasta	Barilla	2 ounces	200	1	0	0	15	42	2	7
Tomato Basil Linguine	Pasta LaBella	2 ounces	200	1	0	0	10	40	2	8

Canned Tomatoes

Choose tomato products that have no added salt. It will help you cut the sodium by hundreds of milligrams. Here are just some examples.

Name	Brand	Serving Size	Calories	Fat	Saturated Fat	Cholesterol	Sodium	Total Carbohydrates	Dietary Fiber	Protein
Tomato Sauce, no salt added	Hunt's	¼ cup	15	0	0	0	15	3	<1	<1
Tomato Paste, no salt added	Hunt's	2 tbsp	25	0	0	0	10	5	<1	1
Tomato Paste, Italian style	Dei Fratelli	¼ cup	20	0	0	0	14	5	1	1

Yogurt

Trying to find the best yogurt is tough! The Breyer's light nonfat ones are low in sugars and also in fat, and they're also the best tasting. They're fortified with calcium and are a good source of protein and potassium.

Name	Brand	Serving Size	Calories	Fat	Saturated Fat	Cholesterol	Sodium	Total Carbohydrates	Dietary Fiber	Protein
Light Lemon Chiffon Nonfat Yogurt	Breyer's	8 ounces	121	0.2	0.2	11.12	101	22.0	0	7.7
Light Key Lime Pie Nonfat Yogurt	Breyer's	8 ounces	124	0.2	0.2	11.12	108	22.7	0	7.7
Light Blueberries n' Cream Nonfat Yogurt	Breyer's	8 ounces	126	0.2	0.2	11.12	102	23.2	0	7.7
Light Peaches n' Cream Nonfat Yogurt	Breyer's	8 ounces	126	0.2	0.2	22.7	102	23.2	0	7.7
Light Raspberries n' Cream Nonfat Yogurt	Breyer's	8 ounces	126	0.2	0.2	22.7	102	23.2	0	7.7
Light Strawberry Nonfat Yogurt	Breyer's	8 ounces	126	0.2	0.2	22.7	102	23.2	0	7.7
Light Strawberry Cheesecake Nonfat Yogurt	Breyer's	8 ounces	126	0.2	0.2	22.7	102	23.2	0	7.7

Nutrition Bars

Whether it's a snack or a meal, sometimes you just need something quick. These are some of the best in terms of their overall nutrition content. Plus, they taste great!

Name	Brand	Serving Size	Calories	Fat	Saturated Fat	Cholesterol	Sodium	Total Carbohydrates	Dietary Fiber	Protein
Gold Bar—Caramel Nut Blast	Balance	1	210	7	4.0	5	90	23	1	15
Yogurt Honey Peanut Bar	Balance	1	200	6	3.0	5	220	22	1	14
Honey Peanut Bar	Balance	1	200	6	3.5	5	220	22	1	14
Chocolate Banana Bar	Balance	1	200	6	4.5	5	190	22	1	14
Oatmeal Raisin Bar	Jenny Craig	1	210	3	0	0	75	35	3	10
Yogurt Peanut Bar	Jenny Craig	1	220	5	3.0	0	270	33	1	10
Milk Chocolate Bar	Jenny Craig	1	210	5	3.5	0	180	33	1	10
Lemon Meringue Bar	Jenny Craig	1	210	5	3.0	0	135	31	0	0

Cookies

Yes, we all have a sweet tooth! Keep some of these on hand in the freezer and enjoy 1 or 2 occasionally.

Name	Brand	Serving Size	Calories	Fat	Saturated Fat	Cholesterol	Sodium	Total Carbohydrates	Dietary Fiber	Protein
Sugar-Free Lemon Crème Cookies	Snackwell's	1	41	1.5	0.3	0	40	7.0	0.1	0.3
Sugar-Free Shortbread Cookies	Snackwell's	1	46	1.5	0.3	2.1	50	7.0	0.1	0.6
Fat-Free Devil's Food Cookie Cakes	Snackwell's	1	55	0.16	0.1	0.1	28	12.4	0.3	0.9

Chapter Twelve

Quick, Yet Gourmet-Tasting Recipes to Help You Eat Away Diabetes

Now for the best part of this book: the food! To preface some very delicious recipes, there is some basic cooking and food information that will make you a real pro in the kitchen. It will also increase your food savvy.

The Diabetes-Friendly Kitchen

One of the secrets to slimming down and living a life free of Type 2 diabetes is culinary savvy—how to whip up gourmet dishes that are big on flavor and slim on calories. Best of all, the ones included here are incredibly easy. I know you have better things to do than labor in the kitchen, such as going for a power walk, playing tennis, or shopping for smaller-sized clothing.

The first and most important trick to healthier cooking when you have diabetes is taking out the fat, especially the saturated fat. Yes, I know, this maneuver can seriously compromise flavor. But I'm going to teach you how to pump up the flavor so that you will prefer your new style of cooking. The only things you'll miss are higher blood sugar readings and your bigger clothing size.

The Ingredients

Lower fat food requires more flavor-enhancing ingredients than higher fat foods because fat is such a great flavor enhancer. There are several ways to build powerfully good taste into recipes from which you remove fat:

- Use a little more herbs and spices than usual. When cooking meat and poultry, forgo all added fat. Instead, add a little more pepper (freshly ground, of course, because it is much more flavorful), an extra shake of low-sodium bouillon granules, fresh herbs, and spices. Using beef bouillon with pork and beef greatly enhances flavor, as does chicken bouillon with chicken and some types of fish. A little-known trick: Use a reduced-sodium variety so that you can use even more without going overboard on the salt.

- Splurge on the best ingredients. Accent your favorite grains, meats, and fish with expensive accessories: Marinate fish or chicken in fresh-squeezed orange juice; use a teaspoon of imported cocoa to make a café mocha; splash double-strength imported vanilla into quick breads.

- Think fresh. Use fresh herbs whenever possible. Fresh basil is far more flavorful than the dried version; ditto for rosemary, mint, and a multitude of others. When fresh is out of the question, use only very recently-purchased dried versions. Most dried herbs lose a significant amount of flavor after six months. Buy small containers of dried herbs and spices, and replace twice yearly.

- Go faux. Learn to use calorie-free extracts instead of the calorie-laden real thing. If you have a Thai recipe that calls for coconut milk, use coconut extract instead. Rum, maple, and many other extracts are necessary pantry staples.

- Replace high-fat ingredients with lower-fat alternatives. For example, use Canadian bacon or turkey bacon for regular bacon in recipes. Low-fat or fat-free cream cheese, sour cream, and yogurt result in fabulous calorie savings.

- Alternatively, use just the right amount of the full-fat version. Do you hate low-fat cheese? Use a scant half ounce of imported Parmesan, feta, Romano, or sharp cheddar in your pasta.

- Toss in some dried fruit. Dried and diced apricots, pineapple, cherries, peaches, and other dried fruits add an entirely new dimension to rice or barley pilaf and to meat.

The Techniques and the Equipment

How you cook is just as important as what you cook when it comes to healthier cooking. Here are some tips on preparing food in your new diabetes-friendly kitchen:

- Treat yourself to the best nonstick cookware and utensils so that you can use less fat with ease.

- Stir-sizzle instead of stir-fry: Use broth instead of oil. This technique works well for meat, poultry, fish, and vegetable dishes. Purchase canned chicken or beef stock (fat-free) or make your own with bouillon granules and water. The latter is preferable because you can make the broth double or triple strength, which enhances the flavor even more. Start with an excellent nonstick pan, coat it with vegetable oil spray or use a scant 1 measured teaspoon of oil, and heat to the desired temperature. Add ingredients and water by the tablespoonful as needed to maintain enough moisture to stir-sizzle. (Note: Many stir-fry recipes call for ¼ to ½ cup of oil, which adds 400 to 800 calories to the recipe.)

- Bake in aluminum foil instead of frying. Add some herbs and a splash of flavored vinegar to a lean chicken breast or fish fillet, wrap in aluminum foil, and bake.

- Toast or roast herbs and nuts to intensify flavor. Place herbs or nuts in a dry nonstick sauté pan and toss over medium heat for three to four minutes until lightly toasted.

- Save the moisture. Cover lean meat very tightly when cooking so that you don't lose the moisture that helps enhance the flavor.

- Make a little fat go a long way: Use the occasional teaspoon of real butter very wisely. Melt a scant teaspoon of butter in a small nonstick sauté pan and add your favorite herb, finely chopped. Sauté over low heat at least five minutes, allowing the herb to soak up the butter and "ripen." Then sprinkle the sautéed herb far and wide on meats, fish, beans, rice, and other grains. You can also extend butter, oil, and mayonnaise with flavored vinegar.

- Coat pans and muffin tins with vegetable oil spray instead of regular oil.
- When making soups and stocks, always allow time to let them chill and then skim the solidified fat off the top.
- Marinate meats, poultry, fish, and vegetables in lower-fat and fat-free marinades to intensify flavor.
- Learn how to make and use yogurt cheese from nonfat and reduced-fat yogurts as a substitute for cream cheese, butter, and sour cream. Buy a yogurt strainer from a kitchen store or make your own with a paper coffee filter and sieve. Line the sieve with the paper filter and place over a bowl that will collect about two cups of liquid. Transfer a quart-size container of fat-free yogurt (plain or flavored) into the sieve. Cover tightly and place in the refrigerator overnight. By morning you will have a thick "cheese." Use as is or stir in herbs, chopped vegetables, or jams.
- Use a food processor to chop, cut, and grate vegetables for recipes. You are more likely to prepare those recipes with lots of veggies if you have some help.
- Have someone else do the work. If you don't like to prepare fresh whole vegetables, buy frozen or already-chopped fresh vegetables found in the produce section. This can be a big help in tossing more veggies into your diet.

The Secret to Using Meat

Yes, you'll be healthier if you choose meat a little less often. I'd like you to go one step further and concentrate on picking leaner cuts of meat. Use the chart on the following page as a guide. Note that a portion is 3 ounces cooked. Rely on your food scale, not your eye!

The Whole Grain Story

It is my hope that you will fall in love with grains as much as I have. Before I tell you a little more about each grain, please note that at the end of this

LEAN CUTS OF MEAT

Each 3-ounce serving of trimmed meat provides 200 calories or less.

Cut of Meat	Calories	Protein (g)	Total Fat (g)	Saturated Fat (g)	Cholesterol (mg)
Pork tenderloin	159	26.0	5.4	1.9	80.0
Canadian bacon	157	20.6	7.0	2.4	49.3
Pork sirloin	181	24.0	8.6	3.0	72.0
Pork center loin	199	22.0	11.5	4.3	68.0
Whole ham	125	19.0	4.9	1.6	44.0
Beef tenderloin	180	24.0	8.5	3.0	71.0
Beef top sirloin	166	26.0	6.0	2.4	75.7
Beef sirloin strip steak	176	24.0	8.0	3.0	64.5
Beef top round	153	27.0	4.2	1.4	71.5
Beef eye round	149	24.7	4.9	1.8	58.7
Beef tip sirloin roast	157	24.0	5.9	2.0	69.0
Beef flank steak	176	23.0	8.6	3.7	57.0
Veal leg	128	24.0	2.9	1.0	87.6
Lamb loin chop	184	25.5	8.3	3.0	81.0
Lamb foreshank	159	26.0	5.0	1.8	88.5
Lamb sirloin leg	174	24.0	7.8	2.8	78.0

section there is a cooking chart for grains. Simplify this job by cooking up large batches and freezing them for up to six months, preferably in half-cup portions. In this way you'll know what you have and can determine how many frozen portions to use in a recipe or for a meal. All uncooked grains should be stored in the refrigerator because they have small amounts of fat (good fats!) and vitamin E, both of which stay fresher in the fridge.

So let's take a look at why I believe you cannot live without whole grains.

Barley

This ancient grain was eaten by Greek athletes to improve athletic prowess. It has a chewy texture and a slightly sweet, nutty flavor.

Barley is loaded with the phytochemicals tocotrienol and lignan. It is also a great source of fiber, especially soluble fiber, as well as vitamin E. This is great not only for controlling diabetes but also for lowering LDL cholesterol (the bad fraction). Barley is also rich in protein, thiamin, niacin, vitamin B$_6$, copper, iron, magnesium, phosphorus, and zinc.

Barley comes in three different forms. Pearled barley, which most people eat, has been milled at least six times, removing all the nutritious bran layers. Medium barley has been milled about three times, making it more nutritious than pearled barley. Hulled barley, the most nutritiously valuable of the three, is the whole grain form. You may also find it as whole barley.

Barley can be used whenever you would use rice; it has far more nutrients and fiber than even brown rice. Use it in soups or stews, make a pilaf with it, or use it instead of rice in a Spanish rice recipe. I have also used some in the muffin recipes in the pages that follow.

Bulgur (also bulgur wheat, or bulghur)

The Romans called it *cerealis,* after Ceres, the goddess of harvest. Ancient Israelites called it *dagan,* a word meaning bursting kernels of grain. These names speak well to how valuable bulgur was in ancient diets and what a rich addition it can be to your diet today. As a form of whole wheat, bulgur retains the wonderfully rich flavor of whole wheat. This Mediterranean staple has a chewy, almost crunchy, yet somewhat tender texture.

Bulgur is rich in protein, dietary fiber (especially insoluble fiber), folate, iron, magnesium, manganese, selenium, phosphorus, and zinc.

Raw bulgur is available in some grocery stores or in a health food store. Made from the whole wheat berry after removing just the inedible hull, it is first steamed, then dried and crushed. Because it is already partially cooked, bulgur cooks up very rapidly, making it easy to use.

Use bulgur in place of rice, as a stand-alone starch dish, as a pilaf, and in cold salads. The most famous Mediterranean dish using bulgur is tabbouleh, which is a combination of bulgur, tomatoes, onion, garlic, lemon juice, and a touch of extra-virgin olive oil (though traditional recipes often have loads of olive oil). Bulgur also makes a great breakfast food: Just cook it up and add some raisins, bananas, and nuts for a hearty, filling breakfast.

Millet

Although used almost exclusively in the United States as animal and bird feed, millet is eaten by a large portion of the world's population, especially disadvantaged third world areas. This bland grain tends to pick up the flavor of the foods it is cooked with. It lends a crunch, giving an interesting texture to many dishes.

While very inexpensive, millet is high in protein, fiber, thiamin, riboflavin, niacin, vitamin B_6, folate, copper, magnesium, phosphorus, and zinc.

Raw millet can be found in some grocery stores and in health food stores.

It is another rice stand-in! Use millet in place of rice in casseroles, soups, muffins, and breads, and also as a breakfast food.

Quinoa (pronounced keen'-wah)

Quinoa looks much like couscous, which is simply a very tiny pasta but is far more nutritious. It cooks similar to rice, expanding to four times its original size. Not actually a grain, quinoa is low in gluten, which is good for those who need a gluten-free diet.

This tiny, bead-shaped grain is incredibly rich in a class of phytochemicals called saponins, which lend a strong taste to quinoa. Most packaging instructions suggest rinsing quinoa before cooking to wash away saponins, but they are best left on the grain to reap the health benefits of this valuable phytochemical. Quinoa is also rich in protein, fiber, thiamin, riboflavin, niacin, vitamin B_6, vitamin E, folate, pantothenic acid, calcium, copper, iron, magnesium, phosphorus, potassium, and zinc. It has more protein than any other grain and has all eight essential amino acids, which is unusual for a plant food.

You can buy quinoa dry in most grocery stores or in health food stores.

Quinoa cooks up like rice, but in half the time. Once cooked, it expands considerably and looks transparent. Use it in soups, salads, and stews as a main dish; it makes a great side dish with the right seasonings. You can stuff it into sweet peppers and poultry. It is very versatile: You can use it as a breakfast food and as a main ingredient topping for cold salads.

WHOLE GRAINS
(per 1 cup cooked)

Grain	Calories	Protein (g)	Fat (g)	Fiber (g)	Rich in These Nutrients
Barley	270	7.42	2.16	13.6	Thiamin, niacin, vitamin B_6, vitamin E, copper, iron, magnesium, manganese, phosphorus, zinc, selenium
Bulgur	151	5.61	0.44	8.19	Niacin, vitamin B_6, folate, pantothenic acid, magnesium, manganese, zinc
Millet	286	8.42	2.40	3.12	Thiamin, riboflavin, niacin, vitamin B_6, folate, iron, magnesium, manganese, phosphorus, zinc
Quinoa	318	11.14	4.93	5.02	Thiamin, riboflavin, niacin, vitamin E, copper, iron, manganese, magnesium, zinc, potassium
White rice	162	3.42	0.26	0.99	Thiamin, riboflavin, niacin,
Wild rice	166	6.54	0.56	2.95	Thiamin, riboflavin, niacin, vitamin B_6, folate, copper, magnesium, manganese, phosphorus, zinc
Brown rice	216	5.05	1.75	3.51	Thiamin, niacin, vitamin B_6, iron, magnesium, manganese, phosphorus, selenium, zinc

Whole Grain Cooking Chart

This chart gives information on preparing one cup of uncooked grain.

Grain	Amount of Water (cups)	Cooking Time	Yield (cups)
Amaranth	4	15 to 20 minutes	2
Barley (whole)	3	1 hour 15 minutes	3½
Brown rice	2	50–60 minutes	3
Buckwheat	2	15 minutes	2½
Bulgur wheat	2	15 to 20 minutes	2½
Cracked wheat	2	25 minutes	2⅓
Millet	3	45 minutes	3½
Quinoa	2	15 minutes	2½
Whole wheat berries	3	2 hours	2⅔
Wild rice	3	1 hour or more	4

Learning About Legumes

I urge you to try all the dried bean and pea—alias legume—recipes in this book. Better yet, I hope that legumes will become your main protein source at lunch and for at least one dinner during each week.

How to Cook Legumes

This chart gives information on preparing one cup of uncooked grain. As with whole grains, you can prepare large batches and freeze them in individual portions or half-cup portions. When sealed well, they keep in the freezer for up to six months.

241

Legume	Amount of Water (cups)	Cooking Time	Yield (cups)
Black beans	4	1½ hours	2
Black-eyed peas	3	1 hour	2
Chickpeas (garbanzo beans)	4	3 hours	2
Great Northern beans	3½	3 hours	2
Kidney beans	3	1½ hours	2
Lentils	3	45 minutes	2¼
Navy beans	3	2½ hours	2
Pinto beans	3	2½ hours	2
Soybeans	4	3 hours or more	2
Split peas	3	45 minutes	2¼

The Wonderful World of Soy

Soy foods make an excellent meat substitute, and therefore a means to reducing the saturated fat in your diet. They are also one of the most versatile legumes. So let's look at them and their many different forms.

Green Vegetable Soybeans (Edamame). These large soybeans are harvested when the beans are still green and sweet tasting. They can be served as a main dish, hot or cold, or even as a snack after boiling for fifteen to twenty minutes. Edamame is found in most grocery stores, fresh in the pod or frozen out of the pod. (Do not eat the pod! The intestinal consequences are disastrous!)

Meat Alternatives (often called meat analogs). Meat alternatives made from soybeans contain soy protein or tofu and other ingredients mixed together to simulate various kinds of meat, such as hamburgers, hot dogs, sausages, and bacon. They are sold frozen, canned, or dried, and are usually used the same way as the foods they replace. With so many different meat alternatives available, the nutritional value varies considerably. They are generally lower in fat, but read the label to be certain.

Miso. This rich, salty condiment is the essence of Japanese cooking. The Japanese make miso soup and use miso to flavor a variety of foods. It is purchased in a smooth paste form made from soybeans, a grain such as rice, salt, and a mold culture; it is then aged in cedar vats for one to three years. Miso should be refrigerated. Use it to make soup, to which you can add small pieces of tofu and vegetables to complete the meal.

Soy Flour. Roasted soybeans are ground into a fine powder that is available in three varieties:

- Natural or full fat, which contains the natural oils found in the soybean
- Defatted, from which the oils have been removed during processing
- Lecithinated, which has had lecithin added to it

All soy flour gives a protein boost to recipes. Defatted soy flour is an even more concentrated source of protein than full-fat soy flour. Although used mainly by the food industry, soy flour can be found in natural foods stores and some supermarkets. Soy flour is gluten-free, so yeast-raised breads made with soy flour are denser in texture. Replace one-fourth to one-third of the flour with soy flour in recipes for muffins, cakes, cookies, pancakes, and quick breads.

Soy Cheese. Soy cheese is made from soy milk. The taste of soy cheese varies greatly by brand, so try more than one if you don't like the first you try. My own personal favorite is Veggie Slices. This brand comes in several flavors—cheddar, mozzarella, and pepper jack—but you might want to try other brands to find one you like.

Soy Sauce. Soy sauce is a dark brown liquid made from fermented soybeans. Soy sauce has a salty taste but is lower in sodium than traditional table salt. Specific types of soy sauce are shoyu, tamari, and teriyaki. Shoyu is a blend of soybeans and wheat. Tamari is made only from soybeans and is a by-product of making miso. Teriyaki can be thicker than other types of soy sauce and includes other ingredients such as sugar, vinegar, and spices.

Soy Yogurt. Made from soy milk, the creamy texture of soy yogurt makes it an easy substitute for sour cream and cream cheese. It can be found in a variety of flavors in most grocery stores and also in health food stores.

Soybeans.   As soybeans mature in the pod, they ripen into a hard, dry bean. Most dried soybeans are yellow, but there are also brown and black varieties. Whole soybeans (an excellent source of protein and dietary fiber) can be cooked and used in sauces, stews, and soups, and as the main topping for salads.

Soy Nuts.   Roasted soy nuts are whole soybeans that have been soaked in water and then baked until browned. They can be found in a variety of flavors, including chocolate-covered. High in protein and isoflavones, soy nuts are similar in texture and flavor to peanuts. They are lower in total fat than most other nuts, and they also have a healthier profile. You can find roasted soy nuts in most grocery stores and in health food stores.

Soy Milk or Soy Beverages.   Soybeans soaked, ground fine, and strained produce a soy milk that is a good substitute for cow's milk. Look for fortified and reduced-fat soy milk in plain, vanilla, and chocolate varieties. A large glass of chocolate soy milk may satisfy a craving for chocolate!

Tofu and Tofu Products.   Also known as soybean curd, tofu is a soft cheeselike food made by curdling fresh hot soy milk with a coagulant. Tofu is a bland product that easily absorbs the flavors of other ingredients with which it is cooked. It is rich in high-quality protein and B vitamins, and is low in sodium. Dense and solid, firm tofu can be cubed to be served in soups, stir-fried, or grilled. Firm tofu is higher in protein, fat, and calcium than other forms. Soft tofu is good for recipes that call for blended tofu. Silken tofu is a creamy product that can be used as a replacement for sour cream in many dip recipes. Look for reduced-fat versions to get the most health benefit from tofu.

Soy Nut Butter.   Made from roasted whole soy nuts, which are then crushed and blended with soy oil and other ingredients, soy nut butter has a slightly nutty taste. It has significantly less fat than peanut butter and provides many nutritional benefits.

Tempeh.   A traditional Indonesian food, tempeh is a chunky, tender soybean cake. Whole soybeans, sometimes mixed with a grain such as rice, are fermented to make this rich cake with a smoky or nutty flavor. It can be sliced like meat and chicken to be used in any stir-fry recipe that calls for either of these. Tempeh can be marinated and grilled, and added to soups, casseroles, and chili or used to make tacos.

Help in the Kitchen

Ever wonder how much uncooked rice it takes to make a cup of cooked rice? What about the number of chocolate wafers you have to crush to yield the one cup of crumbs needed to make a piecrust? Here is the help you need in the kitchen:

Measurements	
Under ⅛ teaspoon	Dash or pinch
1½ teaspoons	½ tablespoon
3 teaspoons	1 tablespoon
1 tablespoon	3 teaspoons
4 tablespoons	¼ cup
5⅓ tablespoons	⅓ cup
8 tablespoons	½ cup
16 tablespoons	1 cup
½ cup	¼ pint
1 cup	½ pint
2 cups	1 pint
4 cups	1 quart
2 tablespoons	1 fluid ounce
3 tablespoons	1 jigger
¼ cup	2 fluid ounces
½ cup	4 fluid ounces
1 cup	8 ounces

(continued)

Foods		
Berries	1 pint	2¼ cups
Butter or margarine	½ stick	¼ cup or 4 tablespoons
Butter or margarine	1 pound	4 sticks or 2 cups
Cream cheese	8 ounces	1 cup
Cottage cheese	8 ounces	1 cup
Parmesan cheese, grated	4 ounces	1¼ cups
Chocolate square	1	1 ounce
Semisweet chocolate pieces	6 ounces	1 cup
Piecrust crumbs	1 cup	19 chocolate wafers 22 vanilla wafers 14 graham cracker squares
Heavy cream	1 cup	2 cups whipped
Dried beans and peas	1 cup	2 cups cooked
Herbs	1 tablespoon fresh	1 teaspoon dried
Elbow macaroni	8 ounces	4 cups cooked
Medium-wide noodles	8 ounces	3¾ cups cooked
Fine noodles	8 ounces	5½ cups cooked
Spaghetti	8 ounces	4 cups cooked
White rice	1 cup uncooked	3 cups cooked
Converted rice	1 cup uncooked	4 cups cooked
Instant rice	1 cup uncooked	1½ cups cooked
Brown rice	1 cup uncooked	3 to 4 cups cooked
Granulated sugar	1 pound	2 cups
Brown sugar, packed	1 pound	2¼ cups
Confectioners' sugar	1 pound	4½ cups

Whole to Sliced Food		
Shredded cabbage	1 small cabbage	4 cups
Grated raw carrot	1 large	1 cup
Sliced carrots	1 pound	2½ cups
Cooked fresh green beans	1 pound	4 cups
Chopped onion	1 large	1 cup
Sliced raw potatoes	4 medium-size potatoes	4 cups
Chopped sweet pepper	1 large	1 cup
Chopped tomato	1 large	1 cup
Canned tomatoes	16-ounce can	2 cups
Sliced apples	4 medium-size apples	4 cups
Mashed banana	3 medium-size bananas	1 cup
Grated lemon rind	1 medium-size lemon	1 teaspoon
Lemon juice	1 medium-size lemon	2 tablespoons
Grated orange rind	1 medium-size orange	4 teaspoons
Orange juice	3 medium-size oranges	1 cup
Sliced peaches	8 medium-size peaches	4 cups
Sliced strawberries	1 pint	2 cups
Soft bread crumbs	2 slices fresh bread	1 cup
Bread cubes	2 slices fresh bread	1 cups
Shredded Swiss or cheddar cheese	8 ounces	2 cups
Egg whites	6 or 7 large eggs	1 cup
Egg white	2 teaspoons egg white powder plus 2 tablespoons water	1
Chopped walnuts or pecans	1 pound shelled	4 cups

Eating away diabetes means starting the day off right—such as with a high fiber muffin or cereal. That's why you'll see several of these recipes right up front in the recipe section. Then, you'll find diabetes-friendly recipes for good eating at all other meals.

Breakfast

Muffins

OAT BRAN APRICOT MUFFINS

Use these muffins for breakfast or for snacks. Don't worry about the big batch; they freeze extremely well for future use. Freezing them the moment they stop steaming seals in the freshness. The pureed pears lend a wonderful taste and texture to these muffins and also cuts the fat, bumping up the fiber considerably. [Makes 36 muffins]

Vegetable oil spray

2 ripe pears

1 cup ground or milled flaxseed

1½ cups oat bran

¾ cup brown Sugar Twin

½ cup packed brown sugar

⅓ cup extra-virgin olive oil

1 cup plain yogurt

1 tablespoon lemon juice

6 egg whites or ½ cup + 1 tbsp. liquid egg white substitute

½ cup wheat germ

1 cup all-purpose flour

1 teaspoon baking soda

1 teaspoon baking powder

2 teaspoons ground cinnamon

½ cup chopped dates

½ cup dried cranberries

20 dried apricots, chopped

Directions

1. Preheat oven to 350 degrees F. Coat 36 muffin cups with vegetable oil spray.

2. Core pears but leave peel on; cut into quarters. Note: If pears are not yet fully ripe, place quartered pears into microwave safe dish with 2–3 tablespoons water and cook on high 3–4 minutes to soften.

3. Place pears in a food processor and puree until smooth.

4. If you purchase whole flaxseed, grind it in a coffee grinder. Many people find it easier to simply purchase ground flaxseed and store it in the refrigerator. Please note that whole flaxseed passes through the body unabsorbed.

5. In a mixing bowl, combine pureed pears, ground flaxseed, oat bran, Sugar Twin, brown sugar, oil, yogurt, lemon juice, and egg whites. Whisk together or beat on low with electric mixer to blend.

6. Add wheat germ, flour, baking soda, baking powder, and cinnamon. Mix with electric mixer or beat with spoon just until dry ingredients are wet.

7. Stir in dates, cranberries, and apricots.

8. Divide mixture among muffin cups.

9. Bake for 20 to 30 minutes, or until a knife inserted in the middle comes out clean.

10. Cool for 5 minutes in pans before removing.

Per Serving Calories: 120, Protein: 4 g, Carbohydrates: 18 g, Fiber: 2.3 g, Fat: 4.1 g, Saturated fat: 0.4 g, % of calories as fat: 30, Cholesterol: 0, Potassium: 148 mg, Sodium: 66 mg, Omega-3 fatty acids: 0

Exchanges Bread/starch: 0.5, Other carbs/sugar: 0.2, Very lean meat/protein: 0.2, Lean meat: 0.1, Fruit: 0.4, Vegetables: 0, Skim milk: 0, Fat: 0.7

CARROT-DATE MUFFINS

These wonderfully rich and colorful muffins are nutritionally packed. Feel free to freeze them for later use. [Serves 24]

Vegetable oil spray

1 cup ground or milled flaxseed

4 carrots

2 ripe pears

½ cup extra-virgin olive oil

6 egg whites or ½ cup + 1 tbsp. liquid egg white substitute

¾ cup packed brown sugar

½ cup brown Sugar Twin

2 teaspoons ground cinnamon

2 teaspoons baking soda

¾ cup toasted wheat germ

1¼ cups all-purpose flour

20 dates, chopped

Directions

1. Preheat oven to 350 degrees F. Coat 24 muffin cups with vegetable oil spray.

2. Grind flaxseed if you have purchased whole flaxseed; otherwise measure ground flaxseed into large mixing bowl.

3. Peel carrots and grate by hand or in a food processor.

4. Remove core and seeds from pears, but leave peel on. Note: If pears are not yet fully ripe, place quartered pears into a microwave safe dish with 2–3 tablespoons water and cook on high 3–4 minutes to soften. Puree pears in food processor.

5. Place ground flaxseed, grated carrots, pureed pears, oil, and egg whites into a large mixing bowl. Beat vigorously by hand or use electric mixer and blend well.

6. Add brown sugar, Sugar Twin, cinnamon, baking soda, wheat germ, and flour.

7. Beat by hand or with electric mixer just until dry ingredients are wet.

8. Stir in chopped dates.

9. Divide mixture among muffin cups.

10. Bake for 20 to 30 minutes, or until a knife inserted in the middle comes out clean.

Per Serving Calories: 174, Protein: 4 g, Carbohydrates: 25 g, Fiber: 2.4 g, Fat: 7.3 g, Saturated fat: 0.8 g, % of calories as fat: 37, Cholesterol: 0, Potassium: 184 mg, Sodium: 131 mg, Omega-3 fatty acids: 0.1 g

Exchanges Bread/starch: 0.5, Other carbs/sugar: 0.4, Very lean meat/protein: 0.1, Lean meat: 0.2, Fruit: 0.5, Vegetables: 0.2, Skim milk: 0, Fat: 1.3

BANANA CHOCOLATE CHIP MUFFINS

In these muffins I've used two secrets that lend body and wonderful flavor and also cut the fat: pureed peaches and flaxseed. My kids think the flaxseed makes them taste just a little nutty, and I agree. These muffins are high in fiber and have enough protein to make a good breakfast accompanied by a glass of milk. The little bit of chocolate satisfies chocolate lovers. The mini chocolate chips make just a little bit go a lot further. Also, these freeze well. [Makes 24 muffins]

Vegetable oil spray

15 ounces canned peach halves with juice, drained

5 ripe bananas

6 egg whites or ½ cup + 1 tbsp. liquid egg white substitute

⅓ cup canola oil or extra-virgin olive oil

¾ cup granulated sugar

¾ cup brown Sugar Twin

½ cup plain nonfat yogurt

1 cup whole wheat flour

1 cup toasted wheat germ

1 cup ground flaxseed

1 teaspoon baking soda

1 teaspoon baking powder

½ teaspoon salt

3 ounces semisweet mini chocolate chips

Directions

1. Preheat oven to 350 degrees F. Coat 24 muffin cups with vegetable oil spray.

2. Puree peaches and bananas in a food processor.

3. Place pureed fruits, egg whites, oil, sugar, Sugar Twin, and yogurt in a mixing bowl. Beat with electric beaters or by hand until smooth.

4. In a separate bowl, mix flour, wheat germ, flaxseed, baking soda, baking powder, and salt.

5. Pour dry ingredients into wet ingredients and beat just until well blended.

6. Stir in chocolate chips.

7. Divide batter among muffin cups.

8. Bake for 20 to 25 minutes, or until a knife inserted in the middle comes out clean.

Per Muffin Calories: 203, Protein: 5 g, Carbohydrates: 33 g, Fiber: 2.8 g, Fat: 7 g, Saturated fat: 1.2 g, % of calories as fat: 30, Cholesterol: 18 mg, Potassium: 177 mg, Sodium: 111 mg, Omega-3 fatty acids: 0

Exchanges Bread/starch: 0.9, Other carbs/sugar: 0.5, Very lean meat/protein: 0, Lean meat: 0.2, Fruit: 0.5, Vegetables: 0, Skim milk: 0, Fat: 1.1

ZUCCHINI FRUITED MUFFINS

These muffins contain cooked barley. Yes, you read correctly! I've used it to cut the oil required and also to give fiber and whole grain goodness. You'll love the interesting texture. If you have a garden, you can grate zucchini when it's plentiful (be sure to include the skin for color, fiber, and nutrients) and freeze it for later use. [Makes 24 muffins]

Vegetable oil spray

2 cups cooked medium barley

1 cup buttermilk

3 tablespoons extra-virgin olive oil

3 tablespoons molasses

6 egg whites or ½ cup + 1 tbsp. liquid egg white substitute

1 tablespoon vanilla extract

2 cups shredded zucchini (including skin)

¾ cup brown Sugar Twin

2 teaspoons baking soda

1 tablespoon ground cinnamon

1½ cups oats (not instant)

1 cup toasted wheat germ

1 cup all-purpose flour

½ cup packed raisins

½ cup dried cranberries

Directions

1. Preheat oven to 350 degrees F. Coat 24 muffin cups with vegetable oil spray.

2. In a large bowl, combine barley, buttermilk, oil, molasses, egg whites, and vanilla. Mix by hand or with a beater until blended.

3. Add shredded zucchini and Sugar Twin, and mix again.

4. In a separate bowl, blend baking soda, cinnamon, oats, wheat germ, and flour.

5. Pour dry ingredients into wet ingredients and stir just until mixed.

6. Add raisins and dried cranberries. Stir gently.

7. Divide batter among muffin cups.

8. Bake for 20 to 30 minutes, or until a knife inserted in the middle comes out clean.

Per Muffin Calories: 146, Protein: 5g, Carbohydrates: 27 g, Fiber: 2.6 g, Fat: 3 g, Saturated fat: 0.5 g, % of calories as fat: 17, Cholesterol: 0, Potassium: 202 mg, Sodium: 134 mg, Omega-3 fatty acids: 0.1 g

Exchanges Bread/starch: 1.1, Other carbs/sugar: 0.1, Very lean meat/protein: 0.1, Lean meat: 0, Fruit: 0.3, Vegetables: 0, Skim milk: 0, Fat: 0.5

THE MOISTEST ZUCCHINI-CARROT MUFFINS

Use this high-fiber and low-fat muffin for breakfast, snacks, or lunches. I've used a better fat, canola oil, and less fat by replacing some of the oil with applesauce. As with other muffins in this chapter, these freeze well for later use. [Makes 24 muffins.]

Vegetable oil spray

3 egg whites or ¼ cup + 1 tbsp. liquid egg white substitute

¼ cup brown sugar

¾ cup brown Sugar Twin

⅓ cup canola oil

¼ cup unsweetened applesauce

1 teaspoon vanilla extract

1 teaspoon ground cinnamon

¾ cup all-purpose white flour

½ cup whole wheat flour

½ cup oat bran

⅓ cup milled flaxseed

1 teaspoon baking soda

1 teaspoon salt

½ teaspoon baking powder

1½ cups shredded or grated zucchini (including skin for color and fiber)

1½ cups grated carrots

Directions

1. Preheat oven to 350 degrees F. Coat 24 muffin cups with vegetable oil spray.

2. In a small bowl, beat egg whites lightly. Add sugar, Sugar Twin, canola oil, applesauce, vanilla, and cinnamon. Whisk together.

3. In a large bowl, mix white flour, whole wheat flour, oat bran, flaxseed, baking soda, salt, and baking powder until thoroughly combined.

4. Pour wet ingredients over dry and stir until just blended.

5. Add zucchini and carrots, and stir well.

6. Divide mixture among muffin cups.

7. Bake for 20 to 30 minutes, or until a knife inserted in the middle comes out clean.

Per Serving Calories: 85, Protein: 2 g, Carbohydrates: 10 g, Fiber: 1.1 g, Fat: 4.2 g, Saturated fat: 0.3 g, % of calories as fat: 42, Cholesterol: 0, Potassium: 98 mg, Sodium: 181 mg, Omega-3 fatty acids: 0.3 g

Exchanges Bread/starch: 0.4, Other carbs/sugar: 0.2, Very lean meat/protein: 0.1, Lean meat: 0.1, Fruit: 0, Vegetables: 0.1, Skim milk: 0, Fat: 0.7

BLUEBERRY MUFFINS

Have these wonderful blueberry muffins for breakfast or for a snack. I've made them appropriately low in calories so that you can enjoy one for snack, which means you can have two for breakfast! I've used cooked cracked wheat for three reasons: for the fiber, for the nutrients, and to reduce the need for oil. The lemon juice tenderizes the muffin and brings out the flavor of the blueberries. You'll love how generous one of these muffins feels, thanks to the great body from the whole wheat products. And they freeze well. [Makes 24 muffins]

Vegetable oil spray
2 cups cooked cracked wheat
1 cup buttermilk
¼ cup extra-virgin olive oil
6 egg whites or ½ cup + 1 tbsp. liquid egg white substitute
1 tablespoon lemon juice

1 tablespoon ground cinnamon
¾ cup brown Sugar Twin
3 tablespoons granulated sugar
2 teaspoons baking soda
1¼ cups wheat germ
1 cup all-purpose flour
3 cups blueberries (fresh or frozen without sugar)

Directions

1. Preheat oven to 350 degrees F. Coat muffin cups with vegetable oil spray.

2. In a large mixing bowl, beat by hand or use an electric mixer to blend cooked cracked wheat, buttermilk, oil, egg whites, lemon juice, and cinnamon.

3. Add Sugar Twin, sugar, baking soda, wheat germ, and flour. Beat just until dry ingredients are wet.

4. Fold in blueberries.

5. Divide mixture among muffin cups.

6. Bake for 20 to 30 minutes, or until a knife inserted in the middle comes out clean (except perhaps for blueberry juice).

Per Serving Calories: 105, Protein: 4 g, Carbohydrates: 16 g, Fiber: 1.9 g, Fat: 3.2 g, Saturated fat: 0.5 g, % of calories as fat: 26, Cholesterol: 0, Potassium: 127 mg, Sodium: 134 mg, Omega-3 fatty acids: 0.1 g

Exchanges Bread/starch: 0.6, Other carbs/sugar: 0.1, Very lean meat/protein: 0.1, Lean meat: 0, Fruit: 0.2, Vegetables: 0, Skim milk: 0, Fat: 0.6

Smoothies

PEANUT BUTTER CHOCOLATE SMOOTHIE

Okay, it's true confession time! I would eat peanut butter chocolate cups much too often if it didn't matter to my weight and my health. This recipe satisfies my craving at either breakfast time or snack time. Afraid of the tofu? Don't be! It lends absolutely no taste but adds the nutrition you need and also a smooth, creamy texture. [Serves 1]

1 tablespoon smooth peanut butter
1 cup chocolate soy milk
4 ounces light firm tofu

Directions

1. Combine all ingredients in a blender and process until smooth.

2. If you like an icier smoothie, add ½ to 1 cup ice cubes.

Per Serving Calories: 267, Protein: 16 g, Carbohydrates: 27 g, Fiber: 0.9 g, Fat: 11.6 g, Saturated fat: 1.8 g, % of calories as fat: 37, Cholesterol: 0, Potassium: 178 mg, Sodium: 171 mg, Omega-3 fatty acids: 0

Exchanges Bread/starch: 0.1, Other carbs/sugar: 0, Very lean meat/protein: 1, Lean meat: 0.4, Fruit: 0, Vegetables: 0, Skim milk: 0, Fat: 1.6

CHOCOLATE RASPBERRY SMOOTHIE

This smoothie reminds me of chocolate raspberry cheesecake except that it's healthier and I can have it for a snack or breakfast or even part of a dinner or lunch. Rest assured you won't taste the tofu; it simply adds great nutrition and rich texture. [Serves 1]

1 cup chocolate soy milk
1 cup frozen unsweetened red raspberries
3 ounces light extra-firm tofu

Directions

Combine all ingredients in a food processor and process until smooth.

Per Serving Calories: 252, Protein: 12 g, Carbohydrates: 55 g, Fiber: 8.3 g, Fat: 2 g, Saturated fat: 0.1 g, % of calories as fat: 6, Cholesterol: 0, Potassium: 235 mg, Sodium: 83 mg, Omega-3 fatty acids: 0.1 g

Exchanges Bread/starch: 0, Other carbs/sugar: 0, Very lean meat/protein: 0.9, Lean meat: 0, Fruit: 1, Vegetables: 0, Skim milk: 2.2, Fat: 0

BANANA CHOCOLATE SMOOTHIE

You're not alone if you've never tried tofu, but remember this key fact: Tofu tastes like nothing but simply picks up the flavors with which it travels. In smoothies, tofu lends a luscious, creamy texture and contributes the protein you need. Add the ice cubes or leave them out depending on how frosty you like your smoothies. [Serves 1]

8 ounces light firm or extra-firm tofu
1 medium ripe banana
1 cup reduced-fat, fortified chocolate soy milk
Ice cubes (optional)

Directions

Combine all ingredients in a blender and process until smooth. This smoothie is thick and creamy, so you might want to enjoy it with a spoon.

Per Serving Calories: 322, Protein: 21 g, Carbohydrates: 53 g, Fiber: 2.8 g, Fat: 4.5 g, Saturated fat: 0.5 g, % of calories as fat: 13, Cholesterol: 0, Potassium: 610 mg, Sodium: 194 mg, Omega-3 fatty acids: 0

Exchanges Bread/starch: 0.2, Other carbs/sugar: 0, Very lean meat/protein: 2, Lean meat: 0, Fruit: 1.9, Vegetables: 0, Skim milk: 0, Fat: 0

Eggs

THREE PEPPERS AND A SPICY CHEESE OMELET

I love to start the day by cooking up an interesting omelet. It is also a great way to get in more veggies at the start of the day. This one has a wonderful concert of textures, from the crisp green peppers to the softer roasted red peppers and, of course, the thick cheese. Leave out the jalapeño peppers or add them depending on your taste buds. [Serves 1]

Vegetable oil spray
2 egg whites, lightly beaten, or ¼ cup liquid egg white substitute
½ cup chopped roasted red peppers from a jar, drained
¼ green bell pepper, chopped
Chopped jalapeño peppers, fresh or from a jar, to taste (optional)
2 ounces 50% reduced-fat cheddar cheese, shredded or grated

Directions

1. Coat a medium-size nonstick skillet with vegetable oil spray and heat over medium heat.

2. Pour in egg whites.

3. Sprinkle with red peppers, green pepper, and jalapeños if desired.

4. Sprinkle with cheese.

5. Cover pan, turn heat to low, and cook until egg whites are congealed and cheese is melted.

Per Serving Calories: 241, Protein: 31 g, Carbohydrates: 10 g, Fiber: 1.3 g, Fat: 9.7 g, Saturated fat: 6.2 g, % of calories as fat: 35, Cholesterol: 30 mg, Potassium: 246 mg, Sodium: 854 mg, Omega-3 fatty acids: 0

Exchanges Bread/starch: 0, Other carbs/sugar: 0, Very lean meat/protein: 1.8, Lean meat: 2.2, Fruit: 0, Vegetables: 1.5, Skim milk: 0, Fat: 0.5

CHEESY ITALIAN SAUSAGE OMELET

If you've never tried veggie ground round (or soy crumbles, found in the freezer case or meat case), this is the time to give it a whirl. Certainly, I would rather have real Italian sausage, but my weight and my blood lipid levels cannot tolerate it. So I worked hard to find something I would enjoy just as much. In fact, because I feel so good about eating it, I love this even more! [Serves 1]

1 teaspoon canola oil
2 ounces veggie ground round
½ cup finely chopped green onions
1 teaspoon Mrs. Dash Classic Italiano or Italian seasoning blend

Vegetable oil spray
2 egg whites, lightly beaten, or ¼ cup liquid egg white substitute
1 ounce 50% reduced-fat cheddar cheese, grated

Directions

1. Heat oil in a medium-size nonstick skillet over medium-high heat.

2. Add veggie ground round, green onions, and Mrs. Dash seasoning. Break up ground round and blend it with onions and seasoning.

3. Sauté until onions are wilted and ground round is slightly browned.

4. Remove mixture from pan and set aside.

5. Wash and dry pan and coat with vegetable oil spray.

6. Heat pan over medium-low heat.

7. Pour in egg whites and allow to set for 3 to 4 minutes.

8. Top egg whites evenly with onion and ground round mixture. Sprinkle cheese on top.

9. Cover pan and cook over low heat until eggs have congealed and cheese has melted, 5 to 8 minutes.

10. Slide from pan and fold in half.

Per Serving Calories: 224, Protein: 28 g, Carbohydrates: 9 g, Fiber: 4 g, Fat: 9.3 g, Saturated fat: 3.7 g, % of calories as fat: 36, Cholesterol: 15 mg, Potassium: 460 mg, Sodium: 547 mg, Omega-3 fatty acids: 0

Exchanges Bread/starch: 0.2, Other carbs/sugar: 0, Very lean meat/protein: 2.3, Lean meat: 1.1, Fruit: 0, Vegetables: 0.8, Skim milk: 0, Fat: 1.1

CINNAMON FRENCH TOAST

French toast the whole family will love! [Serves 1, but multiply to serve others as needed.]

½ cup liquid egg white substitute
½ to 1 teaspoon ground cinnamon
2 teaspoons brown sugar
2 slices whole wheat or oat bran bread
Vegetable oil spray

Directions

1. Blend egg substitute, cinnamon, and brown sugar in a small bowl.

2. Place bread slices in a flat container; pour egg mixture over the top. Flip bread slices to coat other side.

3. While bread soaks up remainder of egg mixture, coat nonstick skillet with vegetable oil spray and heat to medium high.

4. Place bread slices in hot skillet and cook each side until lightly browned.

Per Serving Calories: 277, Protein: 20 g, Carbohydrates: 35 g, Fiber: 4 g, Fat: 6.5 g, Saturated fat: 1.3 g, % of calories as fat: 21, Cholesterol: 1.2 mg, Potassium: 586 mg, Sodium: 520 mg, Omega-3 fatty acids: 0.3 g

Exchanges Bread/starch: 1.7, Other carbs/sugar: 0.5, Very lean meat/protein: 2.1, Fat: 0.6

CHEESY MUSHROOM OMELET WRAP

This is a great recipe to help you learn to love soy cheese. Veggie Slices has the best melting texture and also the best flavor. Mix up the flavors by using a whole wheat wrap or what I call a designer wrap, one of those roasted red pepper ones or a basil pesto variety. [Serves 1]

Vegetable oil spray
4 egg whites, lightly beaten, or ⅓ cup liquid egg white substitute
½ cup chopped green onion
½ cup sliced mushrooms
2 pieces your favorite flavor soy cheese (about 2 ounces)
1 whole wheat wrap

Directions

1. Coat a medium-size nonstick skillet with vegetable oil spray and heat over medium heat.

2. Pour in egg whites.

3. Sprinkle green onion and sliced mushrooms on top.

4. Place soy cheese on top of vegetables.

5. Cover and turn heat to low.

6. Cook until eggs are congealed and cheese is melted.

7. Place wrap on a large plate. Slide eggs from pan onto wrap, roll, and enjoy.

Per Serving Calories: 346, Protein: 29 g, Carbohydrates: 44 g, Fiber: 7.16 g, Fat: 5.8 g, Saturated fat: 0.3 g, % of calories as fat: 15, Cholesterol: 0, Potassium: 569 mg, Sodium: 871 mg, Omega-3 fatty acids: 0

Exchanges Bread/starch: 2.1, Other carbs/sugar: 0, Very lean meat/protein: 2, Lean meat: 0, Fruit: 0, Vegetables: 1.1, Skim milk: 0, Fat: 0

SWEET PEPPER AND CHEDDAR CHEESE SCRAMBLE

My personal trainer was here the day I was developing this recipe, and he nearly turned around and walked out the door when he saw the tofu container. I begged him to try it, and after eating a few bites, he asked if he could finish the whole batch! If you want to make this just for yourself, cut the ingredients in half, but do note that the extras store well in the refrigerator for up to two days. [Serves 2]

2 teaspoons extra-virgin olive oil

½ green bell pepper, chopped

½ red bell pepper, chopped

½ yellow bell pepper, chopped

½ cup chopped onion

12 ounces light firm tofu

3 tablespoons fruit salsa (peach or orange)

2 slices (about 2 ounces) cheddar-flavored soy cheese

Directions

1. Place oil in a medium-size nonstick skillet. Add peppers and onions and cook over medium heat.

2. Add tofu, breaking it up as you sauté peppers.

3. Sauté just until peppers are crisp-tender.

4. Add fruit salsa and soy cheese, and stir well.

5. Turn heat to low, cover, and cook until cheese is melted.

6. Remove cover and scramble mixture.

7. Remove from pan and serve at once. Store extras for later use.

Per Serving Calories: 213, Protein: 18 g, Carbohydrates: 15 g, Fiber: 2.7 g, Fat: 9.2 g, Saturated fat: 0.9 g, % of calories as fat: 38, Cholesterol: 0, Potassium: 426 mg, Sodium: 477 mg, Omega-3 fatty acids: 0

Exchanges Bread/starch: 0.2, Other carbs/sugar: 0, Very lean meat/protein: 1.5, Lean meat: 0, Fruit: 0, Vegetables: 2.2, Skim milk: 0, Fat: 0.9

Oatmeal/Cereal

RAISIN-WALNUT OATMEAL

Try to have oatmeal at least once per week for breakfast. Cooking it with these few simple additions makes it exceptionally delicious. [Serves 1]

⅓ cup old-fashioned oats
1 tablespoon ground cinnamon
1 cup plain, low-fat, fortified soy milk
1 tablespoon raisins
1 tablespoon walnut pieces

Directions

1. In a microwave-safe container, combine oats, cinnamon, soy milk, and raisins. Stir well.

2. Cook on 80% power in microwave for 3 minutes. Stir well and cook on 80% for an additional 3 minutes. Alternatively, place ingredients in a small saucepan and cook on stovetop over low heat for 10 minutes.

3. Sprinkle walnuts on top.

Per Serving Calories: 319, Protein: 16 g, Carbohydrates: 43 g, Fiber: 7.4 g, Fat: 10.3 g, Saturated fat: 1.1 g, % of calories as fat: 28, Cholesterol: 0, Potassium: 677 mg, Sodium: 111 mg, Omega-3 fatty acids: 0.3 g

Exchanges Bread/starch: 2, Other carbs/sugar: 0, Very lean meat/protein: 0.2, Lean meat: 1.1, Fruit: 0.5, Vegetables: 0, Skim milk: 0, Fat: 0.9

BANANA-WALNUT OATMEAL

This version of oatmeal may well be my favorite. It reminds me of banana walnut cake. You can substitute skim milk for the soy milk, but I think you'll love the creamy, rich texture and flavor lent by the soy milk. [Serves 1]

⅓ cup cooked oats
⅔ cup plain, low-fat, fortified soy milk
1 medium banana, sliced
1 tablespoon walnut pieces

Directions

1. In a microwave-safe container, combine oats, soy milk, and banana slices. Stir well.

2. Cook on 80% power in microwave for 3 minutes. Stir well and cook on 80% for an additional 3 minutes. Alternatively, place ingredients in a saucepan and cook on stovetop over low heat.

3. Sprinkle walnuts on top.

Per Serving Calories: 339, Protein: 14 g, Carbohydrates: 54 g, Fiber: 5.9 g, Fat: 9.2 g, Saturated fat: 1.1 g, % of calories as fat: 23, Cholesterol: 0, Potassium: 889 mg, Sodium: 73 mg, Omega-3 fatty acids: 0.3 g

Exchanges Bread/starch: 1.7, Other carbs/sugar: 0, Very lean meat/protein: 0.2, Lean meat: 0.7, Fruit: 1.9, Vegetables: 0, Skim milk: 0, Fat: 0.9

NUTTY IRISH OATMEAL

This version of oatmeal uses the old-fashioned whole grain form of oats, called Irish oats or steel-cut oats. This oatmeal holds up so well once cooked that I often make enough for four breakfasts and just reheat by adding a sprinkle of water and placing it in the microwave. [Serves 2]

½ cup Irish oats
2 cups plain, low-fat, fortified soy milk
1 cup water
1 teaspoon packed brown sugar
½ teaspoon ground cinnamon
2 tablespoons walnut pieces

Directions

1. Combine all ingredients in an electric cooking pot (such as a Crock-Pot) at bedtime. Set on low heat and cook overnight.

2. Stir upon waking and enjoy. The cinnamon will have formed a crunchy crust, which lends to the flavor and texture of this recipe.

3. Alternatively, combine all ingredients in a heavy medium-size saucepan. Place over low heat and simmer for 1 hour, covered, stirring every 15 minutes.

Per Serving Calories: 328, Protein: 14 g, Carbohydrates: 49 g, Fiber: 4.5 g, Fat: 10.6 g, Saturated fat: 1.4 g, % of calories as fat: 28, Cholesterol: 0, Potassium: 454 mg, Sodium: 87 mg, Omega-3 fatty acids: 0.7 g

Exchanges Bread/starch: 3.1, Other carbs/sugar: 0.1, Very lean meat/protein: 0, Lean meat: 0.6, Fruit: 0, Vegetables: 0.1, Skim milk: 0, Fat: 0.9

BLUEBERRIES FOR BREAKFAST

This is so wonderful that you may want to make more than you need for breakfast, and save the extra for snacktimes. Cover and store the extras in the refrigerator up to four days. [Serves 2]

Vegetable oil spray

2 cups unsweetened blueberries, fresh or frozen

2 tablespoons rolled oats

2 tablespoons ground flaxseed

2 tablespoons toasted wheat germ

4 teaspoons trans-fat-free canola margarine

1 tablespoon brown Sugar Twin

2 teaspoons ground cinnamon

1 teaspoon granulated sugar

Directions

1. Heat oven to 350 degrees F.

2. Coat 2 custard cups with vegetable oil spray.

3. Place 1 cup blueberries in the bottom of each cup.

4. In a small bowl, blend the flaxseed and wheat germ.

5. Divide this mixture evenly and sprinkle on the blueberries. Toss gently.

6. Dot each cup with 2 teaspoons margarine.

7. In a small cup or bowl, mix Sugar Twin, cinnamon, and sugar. Divide evenly and sprinkle on top.

8. Place custard cups in oven, uncovered, and bake for 30 to 40 minutes, or until the blueberries bubble.

Per Serving Calories: 238, Protein: 5 g, Carbohydrates: 34 g, Fiber: 7.7 g, Fat: 10.8 g, Saturated fat: 1 g, % of calories as fat: 38, Cholesterol: 0, Potassium: 180 mg, Sodium: 54 mg, Omega-3 fatty acids: 0.2 g

Exchanges Bread/starch: 0.6, Other carbs/sugar: 0.2, Very lean meat/protein: 0, Lean meat: 0.2, Fruit: 1.2, Vegetables: 0, Skim milk: 0, Fat: 1.7

CINNAMON RICE AND RAISINS

My grandmother used to use leftover rice to create what she called "rice and raisins." I've changed her recipe slightly, adding milk to lend protein, and almonds for protein and healthy fat and flavor. Use instant rice at breakfast time or make regular rice the night before and just heat in the morning with a few drops of milk. [Serves 1]

¼ cup instant brown rice
½ cup skim milk
2 tablespoons slivered almonds
2 tablespoons raisins
¼ teaspoon ground cinnamon
Grated orange rind (optional)

Directions

1. In a heavy saucepan, blend rice, milk, almonds, raisins, cinnamon, and grated orange rind if desired.

2. Cover and cook over low heat until rice is fully cooked and soft. The mixture will be slightly soupier than cooked rice.

Per Serving Calories: 294, Protein: 10.4 g, Carbohydrates: 42 g, Fiber: 3.7 g, Fat: 9.7 g, Saturated fat: 0.8 g, % of calories as fat: 29, Cholesterol: 2 mg, Potassium: 487 mg, Sodium: 73 mg, Omega-3 fatty acids: 0

Exchanges Bread/starch: 1.1, Other carbs/sugar: 0, Very lean meat/protein: 0, Lean meat: 0.5, Fruit: 1, Vegetables: 0, Skim milk: 0.5, Fat: 1.7

Main Dishes

Meatless

BLACK BEAN AND ARTICHOKE PITA

This stuffed pita throws together in minutes and is absolutely scrumptious. Notice the fiber in this easy lunch or dinner: 16 grams, with a significant amount of soluble fiber. [Serves 1]

2 tablespoons light Miracle Whip or mayonnaise
½ teaspoon lemon juice
Horseradish as desired
½ cup cooked black beans (canned is okay)
¾ cup canned marinated artichoke hearts
¼ cup chopped green onions
1 small whole wheat pita

Directions

1. In a small bowl, mix together Miracle Whip, lemon juice, and horseradish.

2. Add black beans, artichoke hearts, and green onions, and toss.

3. Cut the top from a whole wheat pita and stuff mixture inside.

Per Serving Calories: 361, Protein: 19 g, Carbohydrates: 56 g, Fiber: 16 g, Fat: 8.9 g, Saturated fat: 1.2 g, % of calories as fat: 21, Cholesterol: 8.3 mg, Potassium: 930 mg, Sodium: 934 mg, Omega-3 fatty acids: 0.1 g

Exchanges Bread/starch: 2.2, Other carbs/sugar: 0.3, Very lean meat/protein: 1, Lean meat: 0, Fruit: 0, Vegetables: 2.9, Skim milk: 0, Fat: 1.4

PASTA PRIMAVERA WITH SPINACH NOODLES

You'll love this fabulously interesting pasta dish, which is as colorful as it is deli-cious. I also love this recipe because it is a help in learning the key to enjoying a large plate of pasta: If you add loads of veggies and intense flavor, the pasta volume is no longer an issue. Gather all the ingredients, cleaning and chopping as neces-sary. The goal is to cook the vegetables while the pasta cooks so that they are done at about the same time. Tossing just-drained hot pasta with rich-tasting ingredients helps the pasta pick up the flavors. [Serves 4]

6 ounces spinach egg noodles, uncooked

1 tablespoon olive oil

3 garlic cloves, peeled and chopped

½ medium red onion, finely chopped

12 ounces raw baby spinach, washed and drained

3 tablespoons lemon juice

1 cup cooked black beans (canned is okay)

4 tomatoes, chopped

8 tablespoons soy Parmesan cheese

Directions

1. Cook pasta according to package directions while working on the vegetables.

2. In a large nonstick pan, heat oil with garlic and onion over low heat for at least 5 minutes.

3. Sauté for at least 5 minutes, one of the tricks to releasing the fabulous flavor of the garlic and onions into the oil.

4. Add spinach, lemon juice, and black beans, and cover.

5. Increase the heat to medium and cook for 5 minutes, just enough for the spinach to wilt but remain brilliant green.

6. When the pasta has finished cooking, drain but do not rinse.

7. Toss hot, drained pasta with hot vegetables.

8. Divide mixture among 4 plates.

9. Top each with chopped tomato and 2 tablespoons Parmesan cheese.

Per Serving Calories: 351, Protein: 20 g, Carbohydrates: 53 g, Fiber: 10.6 g, Fat: 7.9 g, Saturated fat: 1.1 g, % of calories as fat: 20, Cholesterol: 40 mg, Potassium: 1,094 mg, Sodium: 353 mg, Omega-3 fatty acids: 0.24 g

Exchanges Bread/starch: 2.7, Other carbs/sugar: 0, Very lean meat/protein: 0, Lean meat: 0, Fruit: 0, Vegetables: 1.9, Skim milk: 0, Fat: 0.8

THE BEST TACOS

Okay, I'm going to fess up right now: These tacos are meat-free, but I was afraid you wouldn't try them if I called them "vegetarian tacos." They are wonderful because the flavor mimics that of packaged taco seasonings but isn't so outrageously high in sodium. Also, because of the tempeh, the saturated fat is just about nil. Give them a try! [Serves 4]

1 tablespoon canola oil	1 teaspoon paprika
4 garlic cloves, peeled and chopped	⅛ teaspoon cayenne pepper
1 cup chopped green onion (tops and stems)	1 teaspoon ground cumin
½ red bell pepper, chopped	2 teaspoons granulated sugar
½ green bell pepper, chopped	4 flour tortillas
½ yellow bell pepper, chopped	½ cup nonfat sour cream
8 ounces tempeh, crumbled	½ cup salsa
½ teaspoon salt	2 cups chopped romaine lettuce

Directions

1. Heat oil in a large nonstick skillet over low heat. Add garlic and sauté 5 minutes to allow flavor of garlic to release into the oil. Do not burn the garlic.

2. Add green onion, peppers, tempeh, salt, paprika, cayenne, cumin, and sugar. Mix well.

3. Stir-fry, adding 2 to 4 tablespoons water to create some cooking liquid, 5 to 7 minutes, just until all ingredients are hot and well combined in a sauce.

4. Divide mixture among tortillas.

5. Top each tortilla with 1 tablespoon sour cream, 1 tablespoon salsa, and ½ cup lettuce. Roll and eat.

Per Serving Calories: 327, Protein: 19 g, Carbohydrates: 38 g, Fiber: 8.4 g, Fat: 13 g, Saturated fat: 2.6 g, % of calories as fat: 34, Cholesterol: 0, Potassium: 681 mg, Sodium: 509 mg, Omega-3 fatty acids: 0.6 g

Exchanges Bread/starch: 1.6, Other carbs/sugar: 0.1, Very lean meat/protein: 0, Lean meat: 1.1, Fruit: 0, Vegetables: 1.7, Skim milk: 0.3, Fat: 1.3

ENGLISH MUFFIN PIZZA

For lunch time—or anytime—pizza in a snap! [Serves 1, but multiply as necessary]

1 whole wheat English muffin, split in two
2 tablespoons pizza sauce (or ¼ cup reduced-sodium spaghetti sauce)
2 tablespoons finely chopped onion
3 to 5 mushrooms, thinly sliced
⅓ cup shredded part-skim mozzarella cheese

Directions

1. Preheat broiler or toaster oven.

2. Line oven-ready baking sheet with aluminum foil.

3. Place English muffin halves on foil and spread each with pizza sauce.

4. Sprinkle onions, mushrooms, and cheese evenly over both English muffin halves.

5. Place under broiler or in toaster oven just until cheese bubbles and is golden brown.

Per Serving Calories: 328, Protein: 19 g, Carbohydrates: 43 g, Fiber: 7.8 g, Fat: 11 g, Saturated fat: 4.5 g, % of calories as fat: 29, Cholesterol: 22 mg, Potassium: 781 mg, Sodium: 618 mg, Omega-3 fatty acids: 0

Exchanges Bread/starch: 1.7, Other carbs/sugar: 0.6, Lean meat: 1.3, Vegetables: 1.2, Fat: 1

HUMMUS SPINACH WRAP

Hummus is a great way to fit more beans into your diet; this wonderful spread is made from chickpeas. Accented with spinach leaves and grated carrot, this wrap gives you a burst of flavor, as well as great nutrition. Note the high potassium and fiber content of this simply prepared meal. [Serves 1]

1 whole wheat tortilla
⅓ cup hummus (purchased)
2 cups spinach leaves
1 carrot, peeled and grated

Directions

1. Spread hummus over tortilla; top with spinach leaves, sprinkle with carrot.

2. Roll and enjoy.

Per Serving Calories: 490, Protein: 25 g, Carbohydrates: 73 g, Fiber: 18 g, Fat: 14 g, Saturated fat: 1.4 g, % of calories as fat: 26, Cholesterol: 0, Potassium: 2,241 mg, Sodium: 951 mg, Omega-3 fatty acids: 0.3 g

Exchanges Bread/starch: 3.5, Other carbs/sugar: 0, Very lean meat/protein: 0, Lean meat: 0, Fruit: 0, Vegetables: 4.3, Skim milk: 0, Fat: 2.1

STUFFED CABBAGE CASSEROLE

My grandmother and mom always made stuffed cabbages in our Eastern European home. It was a painstaking job that I never learned, nor had the patience for. So, I invented my own version. For a long time I used ground beef, but veggie ground round (a soy protein meat product) works just as well and gives this dish a much better nutrition profile. I hope you enjoy it as much as I do. [Serves 4]

2 tablespoons canola oil

1 leek, cleaned and sliced

1 pound veggie ground round

2 tablespoons very-low-sodium beef bouillon granules

24 ounces Chinese cabbage, shredded

6- to 8-ounce can no-salt-added diced tomatoes

One 29-ounce can no-salt-added tomato sauce

2 tablespoons Mrs. Dash Classic Italiano or Italian seasoning

Directions

1. Preheat oven to 300 degrees F.

2. In a large oven-safe casserole with a lid, heat oil over medium-high heat.

3. Add the sliced leak, ground round, and bouillon. Sauté until the leak is wilted and the ground round is browned.

4. Remove from the heat and add cabbage, tomatoes, tomato sauce, and Mrs. Dash seasoning.

5. Stir well, cover tightly, and bake for 1 hour. Stir twice during the cooking process.

6. Uncover and bake 10 minutes more.

Per Serving Calories: 297, Protein: 31 g, Carbohydrates: 31 g, Fiber: 10.8 g, Fat: 7.7 g, Saturated fat: 1 g, % of calories as fat: 21, Cholesterol: 0, Potassium: 1,779 mg, Sodium: 657 mg, Omega-3 fatty acids: 0.2 g

Exchanges Bread/starch: 0.4, Other carbs/sugar: 0, Very lean meat/protein: 2.7, Lean meat: 0, Fruit: 0, Vegetables: 4.6, Skim milk: 0, Fat: 1.3

PEANUT QUINOA PILAF

Quinoa is one of the grains that we simply don't use often enough. An ancient grain from South America, it is loaded with protein and phytochemicals that may protect us from disease. Serve this dish at room temperature for maximum flavor. [Serves 2]

⅓ cup uncooked quinoa
2 orange spice tea bags
2 tablespoons dry-roasted peanuts
2 tablespoons dried cranberries
½ cup frozen petit peas, thawed
3 baby carrots, thinly sliced

Sauce
1 tablespoon smooth peanut butter
1 tablespoon reduced-sodium soy sauce
1 tablespoon apple cider vinegar
¼ teaspoon ground cumin

Directions

1. Bring ⅔ cup water to a boil in a small saucepan. Add quinoa and tea bags. Lower heat, cover, and let simmer for 15 minutes.

2. Remove from heat, remove tea bags, and flake with a fork.

3. Stir in peanuts, cranberries, peas, and carrots.

4. In a small food processor, combine peanut butter, soy sauce, vinegar, and cumin. Process until smooth. Alternatively, blend all ingredients in a small bowl using a whisk or fork.

5. Pour sauce over salad mixture and toss.

Per Serving Calories: 264, Protein: 10 g, Carbohydrates: 35 g, Fiber: 5.5 g, Fat: 10.5 g, Saturated fat: 1.7 g, % of calories as fat: 35, Cholesterol: 0, Potassium: 419 mg, Sodium: 541 mg, Omega-3 fatty acids: 0.1 g

Exchanges Bread/starch: 1.8, Other carbs/sugar: 0, Very lean meat/protein: 0, Lean meat: 0.5, Fruit: 0.4, Vegetables: 0.3, Skim milk: 0, Fat: 1.4

GARDEN VEGETABLE SAUTÉ WITH MINTED ORANGE QUINOA

Quinoa is a wonderful whole grain food that is loaded with protein as well as minerals and phytochemicals. You'll love this combination of grains and veggies. [Serves 5]

1 tablespoon canola oil

3 small zucchini, cut into small strips

¼ teaspoon minced garlic

1 small red bell pepper, cut into small strips

4 ounces mushrooms, thinly sliced

½ tablespoon chopped fresh basil or ½ teaspoon dried basil leaves

2 tablespoons chopped fresh parsley

1 tablespoon fresh lemon juice

½ teaspoon freshly ground black pepper, or to taste

½ teaspoon salt, or to taste

Minted Orange Quinoa (see recipe on page 275)

Directions

1. Heat oil in a large, heavy skillet. Add zucchini, garlic, pepper, and mushrooms. Sauté over high heat, stirring constantly, about 5 minutes, or until cooked but still crisp.

2. Remove from heat and toss in remaining ingredients.

3. Serve immediately over hot quinoa.

Per Serving Calories: 38, Protein: 1 g, Carbohydrates: 3 g, Fiber: 0.7 g, Fat: 2.9 g, Saturated fat: 0.4 g, % of calories as fat: 62, Cholesterol: 0, Potassium: 143 mg, Sodium: 235 mg, Omega-3 fatty acids: 0

Exchanges Bread/starch: 0, Other carbs/sugar: 0, Very lean meat/protein: 0, Lean meat: 0, Fruit: 0, Vegetables: 0.5, Skim milk: 0, Fat: 0.5

MINTED ORANGE QUINOA

Quinoa is a fabulous grain, rich in protein and phytochemicals, and nearly void of fat. Many people rinse quinoa first, but this washes away the saponins, the phyto-chemical with many health benefits. Quinoa is great hot or cold, for breakfast, lunch, or dinner. As a leftover, this dish is great served cold. [Serves 8]

1 cup raw quinoa

2 cups water

2 spicy orange tea bags

2 teaspoons extra-virgin olive oil

Sauce

3 tablespoons orange juice concentrate

¼ cup fresh mint leaves, packed

3 tablespoons white wine vinegar

⅛ teaspoon salt

Directions

1. Place quinoa, water, tea bags, and oil in a saucepan, and bring to a boil. Reduce heat and simmer for 15 minutes.

2. While the quinoa cooks, make the sauce. Place the orange juice concentrate, mint leaves, vinegar, and salt in a small food processor or blender, and process until the mint leaves are minced.

3. When the quinoa has finished cooking, remove pan from heat and stir in sauce.

Per Serving Calories: 101, Protein: 3 g, Carbohydrates: 17.3 g, Fiber: 1.4 g, Fat: 2.4 g, Saturated fat: 0.3 g, % of calories as fat: 21, Cholesterol: 0, Potassium: 207 mg, Sodium: 42 mg, Omega-3 fatty acids: 0.04 g

Exchanges Bread/starch: 1, Other carbs/sugar: 0, Very lean meat/protein: 0, Lean meat: 0, Fruit: 0.2, Vegetables: 0, Skim milk: 0, Fat: 0.2

WHITE BEAN AND TOMATO PASTA SAUCE

This sauce is loaded with the vegetables your heart demands every day plus a white bean for protein (instead of meat). Using jarred sauce—especially an excellent one—means that you have almost no work to do in the kitchen. [Serves 6]

1 tablespoon olive oil

2 cloves garlic, minced

½ cup chopped red onion

2 cups carrot strips (after peeling the carrot, use the vegetable peeler to create the same type of strips you do when peeling the carrot)

2 cups green zucchini strips (use vegetable peeler to make thin strips using only green portion)

1 cup sliced mushrooms

One 26-ounce jar favorite pasta sauce

1½ cups cooked white kidney beans (cannellini beans)

6 cups cooked spaghetti

Directions

1. Heat oil in a large nonstick skillet over medium heat. Add garlic and red onion, and sauté for 5 minutes.

2. Add carrot strips, zucchini strips, and mushrooms. Sauté an additional 5 minutes, just until vegetables are crisp-tender.

3. Add pasta sauce and beans. Cover and allow mixture to heat through.

4. Serve over cooked spaghetti. One serving is 1 cup pasta and one-sixth of sauce mixture.

Per Serving Calories: 366, Protein: 13 g, Carbohydrates: 66 g, Fiber: 9.2 g, Fat: 5 g, Saturated fat: 1 g, % of calories as fat: 12, Cholesterol: 0, Potassium: 235 mg, Sodium: 774 mg, Omega-3 fatty acids: 0.07 g

Exchanges Bread/starch: 3.2, Other carbs/sugar: 0, Very lean meat/protein: 0.1, Lean meat: 0, Fruit: 0, Vegetables: 0.9, Skim milk: 0, Fat: 0.4

CONFETTI MEAT LOAF

I love meat loaf but don't like all the fat and simple carbs from the bread crumbs or white bread. So I made a few ingredient changes. You will make this again and again. Just don't tell anyone it has veggie ground round and cooked brown rice in it. Remember, you can cook brown rice ahead and freeze it in individual portions to be used in a recipe like this. [Serves 4]

Vegetable oil spray

1 pound veggie ground round

½ cup cooked brown rice

4 egg whites, lightly beaten, or ⅓ cup liquid egg white substitute

½ cup chopped red bell pepper

½ cup chopped green bell pepper

1 cup chopped green onions

2 tablespoons ketchup

Directions

1. Preheat oven to 350 degrees F. Coat a large loaf pan with vegetable oil spray.

2. Place all ingredients in a bowl and mix well with a fork or with your hands.

3. Place in loaf pan and bake for 35–40 minutes.

Per Serving Calories: 195, Protein: 29 g, Carbohydrates: 19 g, Fiber: 7.6 g, Fat: 0.3 g, Saturated fat: 0.1 g, % of calories as fat: 1, Cholesterol: 0, Potassium: 685 mg, Sodium: 668 mg, Omega-3 fatty acids: 0

Exchanges Bread/starch: 0.8, Other carbs/sugar: 0.1, Very lean meat/protein: 3.2, Lean meat: 0, Fruit: 0, Vegetables: 0.9, Skim milk: 0, Fat: 0

PORTOBELLO MUSHROOM CAPS WITH CARAMELIZED ONIONS ON A BED OF QUINOA

While the name makes it appear fancy, don't be concerned that there is a lot of work in this recipe. And don't tell a soul how healthy it is! [Serves 2]

1 tablespoon extra-virgin olive oil

1 clove garlic, chopped

½ medium red onion, thinly sliced and separated into rings

½ teaspoon garlic powder

½ teaspoon oregano

½ teaspoon dried basil

2 tablespoons grated fat-free Parmesan cheese

2 large Portobello mushroom caps, without stems and cleaned

4 ounces soy cheese

1 cup cooked quinoa, hot

Directions

1. Heat oil over medium-low heat in a medium-size nonstick skillet. Add garlic and onion rings. Sprinkle with garlic powder, oregano, and basil. Sauté until onions are softened and slightly browned, about 15 minutes.

2. Sprinkle with cheese and stir well.

3. Remove onions from pan but do not clean pan. Add mushroom caps, top side down, to pan. Fill interior with onions. Add a few drops of water to pan, cover, and steam 5 to 7 minutes, until mushroom caps are tender.

4. Uncover pan and place half of cheese on each mushroom cap. Cover again and heat through just until cheese has melted.

5. Serve each mushroom cap over ½ cup cooked quinoa.

Per Serving Calories: 394, Protein: 24 g, Carbohydrates: 41 g, Fiber: 7 g, Fat: 15.5 g, Saturated fat: 1.2 g, % of calories as fat: 35, Cholesterol: 1 mg, Potassium: 380 mg, Sodium: 568 mg, Omega-3 fatty acids: 0.1 g

Exchanges Bread/starch: 2, Other carbs/sugar: 0, Very lean meat/protein: 0.3, Lean meat: 0, Fruit: 0, Vegetables: 1.5, Skim milk: 0, Fat: 1.4

Beef

GRILLED BEEF FAJITAS

This needs very little introduction. It's a family favorite for my meat-and-potato-loving husband and son. I always cook it in the George Foreman grill, which I just can't live without. [Serves 2]

1 teaspoon extra-virgin olive oil

2 tablespoons balsamic vinegar

2 teaspoons Mrs. Dash Tomato Basil Garlic

2 teaspoons Mrs. Dash Minced Onion Medley

6 ounces beef tenderloin

1 green bell pepper, cut into strips

1 red bell pepper, cut into strips

Vegetable oil spray

2 flour tortillas

2 tablespoons salsa

2 tablespoons fat-free sour cream

Directions

1. In a 9 × 9 glass cake pan, blend oil, vinegar, and Mrs. Dash seasonings to make a marinade.

2. Cut beef into thin strips and place in marinade along with pepper strips.

3. Coat both sides well in marinade. Cover and place in refrigerator at least 1 hour.

4. When ready to cook, heat oven if broiling and coat broiler pan with vegetable oil spray. Or heat outdoor or indoor grill and coat cooking surface lightly with spray.

5. Remove beef strips and pepper strips from marinade and broil or grill until meat is done to your liking. Discard marinade.

6. Place half of cooked meat and vegetables on each flour tortilla. Add 1 tablespoon salsa and 1 tablespoon sour cream.

Per Serving Calories: 311, Protein: 22 g, Carbohydrates: 30 g, Fiber: 3.7 g, Fat: 11.2 g, Saturated fat: 3.4 g, % of calories as fat: 32, Cholesterol: 54 mg, Potassium: 616 mg, Sodium: 229 mg, Omega-3 fatty acids: 0.1 g

Exchanges Bread/starch: 1.1, Other carbs/sugar: 0.1, Very lean meat/protein: 0, Lean meat: 2.5, Fruit: 0, Vegetables: 1.9, Skim milk: 0.1, Fat: 0.7

CLASSIC SPAGHETTI

What's a family menu without the occasional (or frequent) meal of spaghetti? I've made some exceptionally healthy changes to the typical version so that you can enjoy it as frequently as you wish. These include substituting half of the saturated-fat-heavy ground beef with veggie ground round; using no-salt-added tomato sauce; and using salt-free spices. You'll love it—again and again! [Serves 4]

1 teaspoon canola oil

6 roasted garlic cloves (from a jar), chopped (or substitute 2–3 fresh garlic cloves, peeled and minced)

1 medium onion, chopped

4 ounces lean ground beef

4 ounces veggie ground round

One 29-ounce can no-salt-added tomato puree

½ teaspoon salt

1 tablespoon Mrs. Dash Classic Italiano

2 teaspoons Mrs. Dash Extra Spicy

6 ounces spaghetti, uncooked

1 cup chopped fresh parsley for garnish

Directions

1. In a large nonstick skillet, heat oil over medium-high heat. Add garlic, onions, ground beef, and veggie ground round.

2. Sauté until onions are wilted and ground beef and veggie ground round are slightly browned.

3. In a large pot, start water boiling, without salt, for pasta.

4. Add to skillet the tomato puree, salt, and Mrs. Dash seasonings. Cover and simmer for 10 minutes, allowing flavors to release into sauce.

5. While sauce simmers, add pasta to boiling water in pot. Cook pasta according to package directions.

6. Serve one-fourth of sauce over one-fourth of pasta. Garnish with parsley.

Per Serving Calories: 383, Protein: 24 g, Carbohydrates: 59 g, Fiber: 7.8 g, Fat: 6.8 g, Saturated fat: 2 g, % of calories as fat: 15, Cholesterol: 28 mg, Potassium: 1,324 mg, Sodium: 526 mg, Omega-3 fatty acids: 0.16 g

Exchanges Bread/starch: 2.1, Other carbs/sugar: 0, Very lean meat/protein: 0.7, Lean meat: 1.2, Fruit: 0, Vegetables: 4.9, Skim milk: 0, Fat: 0.5

ROASTED KIELBASA AND VEGGIES

Another great recipe for the meat-and-potato lovers in your family, but one that's loaded with nutrition. (You don't have to tell them, though.) This is certainly easy: Throw it in the oven and forget about it. [Serves 4]

Vegetable oil spray

1 pound new potatoes, scrubbed and cut into chunks

1 tablespoon extra-virgin olive oil

1 tablespoon Mrs. Dash Classic Italiano

1 medium onion, peeled and chopped

4 carrots, peeled and thinly sliced

14 ounces low-fat kielbasa, thinly sliced

Directions

1. Preheat oven to 350 degrees F.

2. Coat a large oven-safe casserole with vegetable oil spray.

3. Place potatoes in casserole.

4. Drizzle with oil and sprinkle with Mrs. Dash seasoning. Toss to coat.

5. Add onion, carrots, and kielbasa. Toss again to blend all ingredients.

6. Cover tightly and place in oven. Bake for 45 minutes, or until potatoes and carrots are fork-tender.

Per Serving Calories: 282, Protein: 17 g, Carbohydrates: 42 g, Fiber: 5.1 g, Fat: 6.2 g, Saturated fat: 1.4 g, % of calories as fat: 19, Cholesterol: 35 mg, Potassium: 892 mg, Sodium: 892 mg, Omega-3 fatty acids: 0

Exchanges Bread/starch: 1.7, Other carbs/sugar: 0, Very lean meat/protein: 1.4, Lean meat: 0, Fruit: 0, Vegetables: 2, Skim milk: 0, Fat: 1.1

BARBECUE MEAT LOAF

One of the secrets to enjoying smaller amounts of meat is to spice it up wonderfully. That's what I've done with this meat loaf. Note the addition of oats, which boosts the fiber of this meat dish, especially the soluble fiber that helps control your blood sugars. [Serves 4]

1 pound extra-lean ground beef
¼ cup barbecue sauce
½ cup old-fashioned oats (not quick cooking)
1 cup chopped green onion, tops and bottoms
4 egg whites, beaten lightly, or ⅓ cup liquid egg white substitute

Directions

1. Preheat oven to 350 degrees F.

2. Coat a large loaf pan with vegetable oil spray.

3. In a medium-size bowl, combine ground beef, barbecue sauce, oats, onion, and egg whites.

4. Blend well with a large spoon or with your hands.

5. Place mixture in loaf pan, patting it down evenly.

6. Bake for 35–40 minutes.

Per Serving Calories: 260, Protein: 27 g, Carbohydrates: 11 g, Fiber: 2.3 g, Fat: 11.1 g, Saturated fat: 4.2 g, % of calories as fat: 40, Cholesterol: 41 mg, Potassium: 508 mg, Sodium: 240 mg, Omega-3 fatty acids: 0

Exchanges Bread/starch: 0.5, Other carbs/sugar: 0.1, Very lean meat/protein: 0.2, Lean meat: 3.3, Fruit: 0, Vegetables: 0.4, Skim milk: 0, Fat: 0.2

BEEF STEW

Whether it's a cool day, a day that demands old-fashioned comfort food, or one that requires a one-pot, no-fuss meal, this beef stew fits the bill. The alcohol in the red wine cooks away completely, leaving just the wonderful flavor behind. If you prefer not to use red wine, substitute balsamic vinegar. [Serves 4]

1 tablespoon canola oil

3 cloves garlic, minced

1 pound beef tenderloin, cut into bite-size chunks and all fat removed

2 tablespoons all-purpose flour

2 tablespoons very-low-sodium beef bouillon

1 tablespoon 33% reduced-sodium beef bouillon

1½ cups water

½ –1 teaspoon black pepper

1 large Vidalia onion, cut into chunks

3 large carrots, peeled and sliced

1 pound potatoes with skin, scrubbed and cut into bite-size chunks

¼ cup red wine

One 10-ounce package frozen green beans

Directions

1. In a large, heavy saucepan, heat oil over medium heat. Add garlic and sauté briefly.

2. Add beef chunks and sprinkle with flour. Add both types of beef bouillon, increase heat to high, and brown beef briefly.

3. Lower heat to medium. Add water, pepper, onion, carrots, potatoes, and wine. Cover and simmer, stirring occasionally, until carrots and potatoes are tender, 30 to 45 minutes.

4. Uncover and add green beans. Cover and heat until green beans are piping hot.

Per Serving Calories: 395, Protein: 37 g, Carbohydrates: 34 g, Fiber: 4.8 g, Fat: 10.8 g, Saturated fat: 4 g, % of calories as fat: 25, Cholesterol: 95 mg, Potassium: 1,330 mg, Sodium: 554, Omega-3 fatty acids: 0

Exchanges Bread/starch: 1.2, Other carbs/sugar: 0, Very lean meat/protein: 4.5, Lean meat: 0, Fruit: 0, Vegetables: 1.6, Skim milk: 0, Fat: 1.8

CHECKERBOARD BAKED BEANS

My family absolutely loves baked beans, and I'm always trying to make them just a bit healthier. In this recipe there are two types of legumes (which increases the different number of nutrients), and low-fat kielbasa substitutes for the bacon or sausage usually used. You don't necessarily have to purchase turkey kielbasa for this recipe. Some brands, such as Healthy Choice, have a mixture of beef, turkey, and pork that is quite low in fat. Using ground mustard powder instead of prepared mustard cuts the sodium, as does using no-salt-added tomato sauce. These baked beans freeze well. [Serves 6]

Vegetable oil spray

1½ cups cooked black-eyed peas (canned is okay)

1 cup cooked black beans (canned is okay)

14 ounces low-fat kielbasa

1 large sweet onion, chopped

1 cup no-salt-added tomato sauce

2 teaspoons ground mustard

1 teaspoon chili powder

⅓ cup brown Sugar Twin

1 tablespoon brown sugar

1 tablespoon lemon juice

Directions

1. Preheat oven to 325 degrees F.

2. Coat a large oven-safe casserole with vegetable oil spray.

3. If using canned peas and beans, drain and rinse well. Place in casserole dish.

4. Slice kielbasa thinly and then cut slices into quarters. Add to casserole.

5. Add onion, tomato sauce, mustard, chili powder, Sugar Twin, brown sugar, and lemon juice. Mix well.

6. Place casserole in oven, uncovered, and bake for 45 minutes, stirring once or twice.

Per Serving (about ¾ cup) Calories: 376, Protein: 26 g, Carbohydrates: 61 g, Fiber: 10.5 g, Fat: 3.1 g, Saturated fat: 0.9 g, % of calories as fat: 8, Cholesterol: 24 mg, Potassium: 1,003 mg, Sodium: 602 mg, Omega-3 fatty acids: 0.2 g

Exchanges Bread/starch: 3.5, Other carbs/sugar: 0.2, Very lean meat/protein: 1, Lean meat: 0, Fruit: 0, Vegetables: 1, Skim milk: 0, Fat: 0.3

Poultry

OVEN-FRIED CHICKEN

You're going to be absolutely amazed at how great this oven-fried chicken is—made with high-fiber cereal. I hope my son doesn't read this part of the book, as he has no clue that his favorite fried chicken is made this way. Give it a try—at least once! [Serves 2]

Vegetable oil spray

1 cup Fiber One cereal

2 teaspoons 33% reduced-sodium chicken bouillon

1 tablespoon very-low-sodium chicken bouillon

Black pepper to taste

1 teaspoon canola oil

3 tablespoons egg substitute, or 2 egg whites, slightly beaten

8 ounces boneless, skinless chicken breast

Directions

1. Preheat oven to 350 degrees F. Coat a cookie sheet with vegetable oil spray.

2. In a food processor, combine cereal, both types of bouillon, and pepper. Process until it is fine "meal." Alternatively, crush the cereal with a rolling pin or other means. Be sure it is exceptionally fine. Place in a small, flat container.

3. In another small, flat container, whisk together the oil and egg substitute.

4. Cut chicken into strips and dip into egg-oil mixture. Then dredge in cereal meal, coating each strip well.

5. Place each strip on the cookie sheet and coat tops of strips with vegetable oil spray.

6. Bake for 30 minutes.

Per Serving Calories: 285, Protein: 38.5 g, Carbohydrates: 24.2 g, Fiber: 14.3 g, Fat: 7.3 g, Saturated fat: 1.4 g, % of calories as fat: 21, Cholesterol: 87.6 mg, Potassium: 507 mg, Sodium: 856 mg, Omega-3 fatty acids: 0.32 g

Exchanges Bread/starch: 0.8, Other carbs/sugar: 0, Very lean meat/protein: 5, Lean meat: 0, Fruit: 0, Vegetables: 0, Skim milk: 0, Fat: 0.7

TOMATO-BARLEY CHICKEN STEW

This one-pot meal is very easy to prepare and loaded with a symphony of flavors you'll love. [Serves 4]

1 tablespoon canola oil

3 cloves garlic, minced

1 white onion, chopped

1 pound boneless, skinless chicken breast, cut into chunks

4 teaspoons 33% reduced-sodium chicken bouillon granules

One 15-ounce can no-salt-added tomato puree

¾ cup uncooked barley

3 cups water

2 teaspoons Mrs. Dash Classic Italiano or Italian seasoning

2 cups sun-dried tomatoes (dry pack, not packed in oil)

8 ounces snow peas, cleaned

Directions

1. Heat oil in a large, heavy pot over medium heat. Add garlic and onion. Sauté for 5 minutes, allowing flavors to release into oil. Do not burn the garlic.

2. Add chicken and bouillon granules. Increase heat to high and brown for 5 minutes.

3. Reduce heat to medium-low. Add tomato puree, barley, water, Mrs. Dash seasoning, and tomatoes.

4. Cover and simmer barley according to package directions, generally 30 to 45 minutes, stirring occasionally.

5. Remove cover, add snow peas, and stir well.

6. Cover and steam for 5 minutes. The snow peas will still be crunchy.

Per Serving Calories: 454, Protein: 35 g, Carbohydrates: 62 g, Fiber: 13.3 g, Fat: 7.6 g, Saturated fat: 1.3 g, % of calories as fat: 15, Cholesterol: 63 mg, Potassium: 929 mg, Sodium: 1,118 mg, Omega-3 fatty acids: 0.4 g

Exchanges Bread/starch: 2, Other carbs/sugar: 0, Very lean meat/protein: 3.2, Lean meat: 0, Fruit: 0, Vegetables: 5.4, Skim milk: 0, Fat: 1

CREAMY CHICKEN AND RICE

This is a wonderfully healthy version of a venerable comfort food. The wild rice is well worth the time and money, so please give it a try. [Serves 4]

1 tablespoon extra-virgin olive oil

1 yellow onion, chopped

½ cup uncooked wild rice

2 cups water

2 teaspoons low-sodium chicken bouillon granules

½ cup uncooked brown rice (not quick cooking)

2 cans low-sodium cream of mushroom soup

1 pound boneless, skinless chicken breast

One 10-ounce package frozen broccoli

Directions

1. In a large, heavy pot, heat oil over medium-low heat. Add onion and sauté until slightly wilted.

2. Add wild rice, water, bouillon granules, and brown rice. Cover tightly and simmer for 30 minutes.

3. Uncover and stir in soup.

4. Place chicken on top of rice mixture. Cover and simmer 30 minutes more.

5. Uncover, remove chicken to a plate, and stir broccoli into rice. Replace chicken on top of rice-broccoli mixture.

6. Cover and steam just until broccoli is heated through.

Per Serving Calories: 520, Protein: 44 g, Carbohydrates: 51 g, Fiber: 6.6 g, Fat: 15.6 g, Saturated fat: 3.8 g, % of calories as fat: 27, Cholesterol: 106 mg, Potassium: 660 mg, Sodium: 134 mg, Omega-3 fatty acids: 0.3 g

Exchanges Bread/starch: 2.7, Other carbs/sugar: 0, Very lean meat/protein: 5, Lean meat: 0, Fruit: 0, Vegetables: 1.3, Skim milk: 0, Fat: 2.2

HERBED CHICKEN AND PASTA

Casseroles are a big hit in our household, but using the canned soup or packaged seasoning mix became less of an option when I had to cut back on sodium. Non-sodium seasoning and a few more creative ingredients solved that problem and also satisfied my fussy family. [Serves 2]

2 teaspoons canola oil

2 garlic cloves, minced

8 ounces boneless, skinless chicken breast, cut into cubes

1 carrot, peeled and very thinly sliced

1 teaspoon 33% reduced-sodium chicken bouillon granules

2 tablespoons very-low-sodium chicken bouillon

⅛ to ¼ teaspoon ground black pepper

2 tablespoons Mrs. Dash Classic Italiano

8 ounces mushrooms, sliced

One 10-ounce package frozen asparagus spears, thawed

1 can condensed low-sodium cream of mushroom soup

2 tablespoons lemon juice

2 cups cooked rotini pasta noodles

2 tablespoons grated fat-free Parmesan cheese

Directions

1. In an extra-large nonstick skillet or electric fry pan, heat oil over low heat. Add garlic and sauté for 5 minutes, allowing garlic flavor to release into oil. Do not burn garlic.

2. Increase heat to medium-high. Add chicken and carrot slices. Sprinkle with both types of chicken bouillon, pepper, and Mrs. Dash seasoning.

3. Add ¼ cup water and stir-sizzle, as I call this method of lower fat cooking, for 5 minutes, or until chicken and carrots are slightly browned.

4. Lower heat to medium-low. Add mushrooms, asparagus, mushroom soup, and lemon juice. Blend well.

5. Cover and simmer for 20 minutes. Uncover and fold in cooked pasta.

6. Divide chicken-pasta mixture between 2 plates. Sprinkle each with 1 tablespoon cheese.

Per Serving Calories: 488, Protein: 37 g, Carbohydrates: 38 g, Fiber: 4 g, Fat: 21.7 g, Saturated fat: 4.5 g, % of calories as fat: 39, Cholesterol: 66 mg, Potassium: 696 mg, Sodium: 519 mg, Omega-3 fatty acids: 0.8 g

Exchanges Bread/starch: 1.6, Other carbs/sugar: 0, Very lean meat/protein: 3.5, Lean meat: 0, Fruit: 0.1, Vegetables: 1.9, Skim milk: 0, Fat: 3.7

SESAME GINGER CHICKEN STIR-FRY

There is something almost magical about the combined flavors of sesame, garlic, ginger, and soy sauce. This stir-fry is also beautiful to the eye, which means you are satisfied at first glance! [Serves 2]

2 teaspoons sesame oil

2 cloves garlic, minced

2 tablespoons minced fresh ginger

3 green onions, finely chopped

8 ounces boneless, skinless chicken breast, cut into thin strips

¼ teaspoon black pepper

2 tablespoons reduced-sodium soy sauce

1 teaspoon sugar

2 cups snow peas, cleaned

2 cups frozen carrot slices, defrosted

1 red bell pepper, chopped

½ cup chopped fresh cilantro

Directions

1. Heat oil in a large nonstick skillet over medium heat with garlic and ginger. Sauté for 2 to 3 minutes.

2. Add onions, chicken, pepper, and a few teaspoons of water.

3. Increase heat and stir-sizzle about 5 minutes, until chicken is browned.

4. Reduce heat to medium. Add soy sauce, sugar, snow peas, carrot slices, and bell pepper. Cover and steam about 5 minutes. The vegetables will still be crisp-tender except for the carrot slices.

5. Remove from heat and stir in cilantro.

Per Serving Calories: 350, Protein: 31 g, Carbohydrates: 38 g, Fiber: 12.1 g, Fat: 8.4 g, Saturated fat: 1.7 g, % of calories as fat: 21, Cholesterol: 63 mg, Potassium: 1,076 mg, Sodium: 683 mg, Omega-3 fatty acids: 0.1 g

Exchanges Bread/starch: 1, Other carbs/sugar: 0.1, Very lean meat/protein: 3.2, Lean meat: 0, Fruit: 0, Vegetables: 3.3, Skim milk: 0, Fat: 1.1

TURKEY TOMATO WRAP

This is a wonderfully delicious wrap for a quick lunch or dinner. Be creative with the wraps, such as using a roasted red pepper or pesto wrap. [Serves 1]

1 tablespoon light mayonnaise
1 carrot, grated
1 tomato, chopped
1 whole wheat wrap
3 ounces cooked, boneless, skinless turkey breast, thinly sliced
1 cup chopped raw spinach

Directions

1. Blend the light mayonnaise into the grated carrot. Stir in tomatoes.

2. Spread on the whole wheat wrap. Arrange the turkey slices on top.

3. Add spinach leaves, roll, and eat.

Per Serving Calories: 299, Protein: 31 g, Carbohydrates: 34 g, Fiber: 5.7 g, Fat: 6.4 g, Saturated fat: 1.1 g, % of calories as fat: 18, Cholesterol: 76 mg, Potassium: 985 mg, Sodium: 407 mg, Omega-3 fatty acids: 0.1 g

Exchanges Bread/starch: 0.9, Other carbs/sugar: 0.1, Very lean meat/protein: 3.3, Lean meat: 0, Fruit: 0, Vegetables: 2.4, Skim milk: 0, Fat: 1

Pork

PORK AND PEAR STEW

This is my absolute favorite pork dish. It's so easy but so very rich in flavor. Like other dishes that use alcohol, the alcohol cooks off and leaves a fabulously rich flavor behind. [Serves 4]

1 teaspoon canola oil

1 red onion, chopped

1 pound lean pork roast sirloin, trimmed of fat and cut into bite-size pieces

4 just-ripe pears, sliced into quarters, core removed (but skin left on), and cut lengthwise into thin slices

¾ cup pear nectar

1 tablespoon dried thyme

¼ cup plus 2 tablespoons sherry

½ cup nonfat sour cream

Directions

1. Heat oil with onion in a large nonstick skillet over medium heat. Sauté onion just until wilted.

2. Increase heat to medium-high. Add pork and sauté until browned, 5 to 7 minutes.

3. Reduce heat to medium-low. Add pears, pear nectar, thyme, and sherry.

4. Simmer, uncovered, until pears are fork-tender and liquid has reduced, 20 to 30 minutes.

5. Stir in sour cream.

Per Serving Calories: 341, Protein: 28 g, Carbohydrates: 28 g, Fiber: 5.6 g, Fat: 11.4 g, Saturated fat: 3.4 g, % of calories as fat: 29, Cholesterol: 73 mg, Potassium: 605 mg, Sodium: 222 mg, Omega-3 fatty acids: 0

Exchanges Bread/starch: 0, Other carbs/sugar: 0, Very lean meat/protein: 0, Lean meat: 3.4, Fruit: 1.3, Vegetables: 0.5, Skim milk: 0.3, Fat: 0.9

CREAMY PORK AND PARSNIPS

You'll love this easy stovetop casserole—and your body will love the great nutrition and fiber. [Serves 4]

Vegetable oil spray

1 pound lean pork tenderloin, cut into chunks

2 onions, chopped

2 teaspoons 33% reduced-sodium beef bouillon granules

1 can ready-to-serve low-sodium cream of mushroom soup

4 parsnips, peeled and thinly sliced

4 carrots, peeled and thinly sliced

Black pepper to taste

Directions

1. Coat a large nonstick skillet with vegetable oil spray and heat over medium-high heat. Add pork and brown on all sides.

2. Reduce heat to a simmer. Add onions, bouillon granules, soup, parsnips, and carrots. Stir well.

3. Cover and simmer about 30 minutes, until carrots and parsnips are fork-tender and pork is cooked through. Add pepper if desired.

Per Serving Calories: 377, Protein: 29 g, Carbohydrates: 50 g, Fiber: 10.1 g, Fat: 8.1 g, Saturated fat: 2.5 g, % of calories as fat: 23, Cholesterol: 68 mg, Potassium: 1,375 mg, Sodium: 798 mg, Omega-3 fatty acids: 0

Exchanges Bread/starch: 0.3, Other carbs/sugar: 0, Very lean meat/protein: 3.4, Lean meat: 0, Fruit: 0, Vegetables: 8.6, Skim milk: 0, Fat: 1.5

SAGE-SIMMERED PORK CHOPS

Sage highlights the fabulous flavor of pork. This easy recipe makes for a quick, yet delicious gourmet dinner. [Serves 4]

1 tablespoon canola oil, divided

2 small onions, chopped

8 ounces mushrooms, sliced

2 teaspoons beef bouillon granules

2 teaspoons very-low-sodium beef bouillon granules

4 tablespoons all-purpose flour

1 teaspoon ground sage

⅓ cup liquid egg white substitute, or 4 egg whites, lightly beaten

4 pork chops, all visible fat removed

Directions

1. Heat 1 teaspoon oil in a large nonstick skillet over medium heat. Add onions and mushrooms, and sauté until onions are wilted. Remove from pan but do not wash pan. Set pan aside until ready to cook pork chops.

2. Meanwhile, blend both types of bouillon granules, flour, and sage in a small, flat container.

3. Pour the egg substitute into another small, flat container.

4. Dip each pork chop first in egg substitute and then in flour mixture.

5. Add remaining 2 teaspoons oil to pan and heat to medium-high

6. Place pork chops in pan and brown on each side; add 1–2 tablespoons water as needed to stir-sizzle.

7. Reduce heat to a simmer and cover pan tightly. Cook pork chops thoroughly.

8. Open pan and place sautéed onions and mushrooms on top of pork chops. Cover and steam briefly.

Per Serving Calories: 233, Protein: 24 g, Carbohydrates: 12 g, Fiber: 3 g, Fat: 9.3 g, Saturated fat: 2.3 g, % of calories as fat: 37, Cholesterol: 52 mg, Potassium: 366 mg, Sodium: 533 mg, Omega-3 fatty acids: 0.4 g

Exchanges Bread/starch: 0.4, Other carbs/sugar: 0, Very lean meat/protein: 3, Lean meat: 0, Fruit: 0, Vegetables: 1.2, Skim milk: 0, Fat: 1.5

PORK TENDERLOIN STIR-FRY

This recipe is a great example of using meat as a garnish rather than the focal point of the meal. This stir-fry marries some unexpected ingredients for an explosion of flavor. [Serves 2]

1 teaspoon sesame oil

2 cloves garlic, peeled and minced

½ medium onion, chopped

8 ounces lean pork tenderloin, cut into strips

½ teaspoon ground black pepper

1 teaspoon ground ginger

1 pound snow peas, cleaned

8-ounce can water chestnuts, drained

3 tablespoons orange marmalade

2 tablespoons low-sodium soy sauce

1 tablespoon cornstarch

Directions

1. Heat oil in a large nonstick skillet over medium heat with garlic and onion. Sauté 5 minutes, until onions are wilted. Do not burn garlic.

2. Increase heat to high and add pork, pepper, and ginger. Brown briefly, 3 or 4 minutes.

3. Reduce heat to medium. Add snow peas and water chestnuts. Sauté until meat is cooked through. Snow peas will still be crisp-tender.

4. In a small bowl, whisk together marmalade, soy sauce, and cornstarch.

5. Increase heat to medium-high. While gently stirring vegetables and meat, slowly pour sauce over them. Stir constantly until sauce thickens, then remove at once from heat.

Per Serving Calories: 501, Protein: 43 g, Carbohydrates: 60 g, Fiber: 12.6 g, Fat: 10.5 g, Saturated fat: 3 g, % of calories as fat: 19, Cholesterol: 107 mg, Potassium: 1,079 mg, Sodium: 649 mg, Omega-3 fatty acids: 0.1 g

Exchanges Bread/starch: 1.4, Other carbs/sugar: 1.2, Very lean meat/protein: 5, Lean meat: 0, Fruit: 0, Vegetables: 3.2, Skim milk: 0, Fat: 1.4

Soups

LENTIL STEW

This vegetarian meal will convince you to add other vegetarian meals to your regular eating plan. It is an excellent example to show that tofu has no flavor but simply picks up flavor from what you pair it with. Here the tofu is used as the thickening agent, and it lends a fabulous creamy texture. [Serves 2]

1 tablespoon extra-virgin olive oil

4 shallots, cleaned and sliced

3 tablespoons all-purpose flour

2 teaspoons vegetable bouillon or paste

Freshly ground black pepper to taste

½ cup uncooked lentils (can use orange or green lentils)

2 large carrots (about 12 ounces), peeled and thinly sliced

2 celery stalks, cleaned and thinly sliced

8 ounces mushrooms, sliced

6 ounces light extra-firm tofu

Directions

1. Heat oil in a large, heavy kettle over medium-low heat with shallots, flour, bouillon, and pepper. Sauté until onions are wilted.

2. Add lentils, carrots, celery, and 2 cups water. Cover tightly and simmer for 30 minutes.

3. Add mushrooms and simmer, covered, 15 minutes more.

4. Meanwhile, puree tofu in a food processor or blend with an electric mixer until smooth.

5. Stir tofu into lentil mixture and simmer an additional 10 minutes, uncovered.

Per Serving Calories: 418, Protein: 27 g, Carbohydrates: 59 g, Fiber: 18.6 g, Fat: 8.6 g, Saturated fat: 1.2 g, % of calories as fat: 18, Cholesterol: 0, Potassium: 890 mg, Sodium: 735 mg, Omega-3 fatty acids: 0.1 g

Exchanges Bread/starch: 2.4, Other carbs/sugar: 0, Very lean meat/protein: 1.3, Lean meat: 0, Fruit: 0, Vegetables: 3.9, Skim milk: 0, Fat: 1.4

CREAM OF MUSHROOM AND BARLEY SOUP

My mom taught me to love the combined flavors of barley and mushrooms. This re-creation of one of my favorite soups is wonderfully delicious and yet has lower sodium and very low fat. In addition, you get the benefit of soluble-fiber-rich barley. [Serves 4]

2 tablespoons extra-virgin olive oil

1 cup chopped green onions

1 pound mushrooms, cleaned and sliced

2 tablespoons water

2 teaspoons vegetable bouillon

2 tablespoons Mrs. Dash Classic Italiano or Italian seasoning

2 cups skim milk, divided

2 teaspoons cornstarch

12 ounces light, firm tofu

1 cup medium barley, cooked

Directions

1. In a large, heavy kettle, heat oil over medium-low heat with green onions. Sauté until onions are wilted.

2. Add mushrooms, water, bouillon, and Mrs. Dash seasoning. Cover and simmer until mushrooms are fork-tender.

3. Meanwhile, place in a food processor 2 tablespoons skim milk, the cornstarch, and tofu. Process until smooth.

4. Pour mixture into cooked mushrooms along with remaining skim milk. Whisk until mixture has warmed and thickened slightly.

5. Stir in cooked barley; cover and allow barley to heat through.

Per Serving Calories: 294, Protein: 16 g, Carbohydrates: 43 g, Fiber: 4.5 g, Fat: 8.7 g, Saturated fat: 1.5 g, % of calories as fat: 25, Cholesterol: 2 mg, Potassium: 785 mg, Sodium: 425 mg, Omega-3 fatty acids: 0.1 g

Exchanges Bread/starch: 1.6, Other carbs/sugar: 0, Very lean meat/protein: 0.8, Lean meat: 0, Fruit: 0, Vegetables: 1.4, Skim milk: 0.5, Fat: 1.4

BLACK BEAN SOUP WITH CILANTRO

This interesting soup is definitely "company" food because it is gourmet in quality. But it's so easy that you'll make it for yourself again and again. [Serves 4]

1 tablespoon olive oil

3 garlic cloves, chopped

1 pound arugula, washed

4 tablespoons lime juice

1 tablespoon ground cilantro

1 cup sun-dried tomatoes

One 15-ounce can refried black beans

1 cup soy milk

½ cup fat-free croutons for garnish

½ cup chopped fresh cilantro for garnish

Directions

1. In a large, heavy kettle, heat oil over low heat with garlic. Stir-fry for 3 to 5 minutes to fully release the garlic flavor.

2. Add arugula, lime juice, and ground cilantro. Cover and let steam 5 to 7 minutes, or until arugula is soft.

3. Remove from heat. Place mixture with cooking liquid into a food processor and process until smooth.

4. Return pureed mixture to kettle. Add tomatoes, beans, and soy milk. Whisk until smooth.

5. Cover and cook over low heat 5 to 10 minutes, or until tomatoes plump up slightly.

6. Garnish each bowl of soup with croutons and fresh cilantro.

Per Serving Calories: 253, Protein: 13 g, Carbohydrates: 36 g, Fiber: 9.2 g, Fat: 8.3 g, Saturated fat: 1 g, % of calories as fat: 27, Cholesterol: 0, Potassium: 1,021 mg, Sodium: 706 mg, Omega-3 fatty acids: 0.23 g

Exchanges Bread/starch: 0.6, Other carbs/sugar: 0, Very lean meat/protein: 0.3, Lean meat: 0.3, Fruit: 0.1, Vegetables: 2.2, Skim milk: 0, Fat: 0.8

CREAM OF SPINACH AND MUSHROOM SOUP

This heartwarming soup is also heart-healthfully fabulous. Best of all, it's so easy to prepare. [Serves 2]

1 tablespoon extra-virgin olive oil

1 leek, cleaned and thinly sliced

8 ounces mushrooms, cleaned and sliced

One 10-ounce package frozen spinach, thawed

1 cup low-fat cottage cheese

1 cup plain low-fat, fortified soy milk or skim milk

Directions

1. In a medium, heavy kettle, heat oil over low heat with leek. Sauté about 5 minutes, until leek is wilted.

2. Add mushrooms and spinach, and stir well. Cover and simmer until mushrooms are fork-tender.

3. Meanwhile, puree cottage cheese in a food processor until smooth.

4. Once mushrooms are cooked, stir in cottage cheese and soy milk until mixture is creamy smooth and hot.

Per Serving Calories: 283, Protein: 27 g, Carbohydrates: 25 g, Fiber: 5.8 g, Fat: 11.2 g, Saturated fat: 2.3 g, % of calories as fat: 33, Cholesterol: 15 mg, Potassium: 1,615 mg, Sodium: 555 mg, Omega-3 fatty acids: 0.3 g

Exchanges Bread/starch: 0.4, Other carbs/sugar: 0.3, Very lean meat/protein: 2, Lean meat: 0.5, Fruit: 0, Vegetables: 2.9, Skim milk: 0, Fat: 1.3

GINGER-LENTIL-BARLEY SOUP

This recipe was one of those culinary experimentations that turned out extremely well. This recipe is also a great way to get in some green tea even if you have never liked it! This has now become my favorite soup, and I hope you like it, too. [Serves 4]

1 tablespoon extra-virgin olive oil	2 large carrots, peeled and thinly sliced
2 cloves garlic, peeled and sliced	4 green tea bags
½ red onion, peeled and chopped	One 1-inch piece ginger, finely diced
4 teaspoons vegetable bouillon	3 small green zucchini, with peel on and washed
½ cup dry lentils	½ medium red bell pepper
½ cup medium barley	½ medium green bell pepper
6 cups water	

Directions

1. Heat oil in a heavy kettle over low heat with garlic and onion. Sauté for 5 minutes to release flavor into oil.

2. Add bouillon, lentils, barley, water, carrots, tea bags, and ginger. Cover tightly and simmer for 30 minutes.

3. Meanwhile, prepare vegetables: Slice the zucchini and then quarter the slices. Chop the bell peppers.

4. After lentils and barley are cooked (about 30 minutes), add zucchini. Cover and simmer 30 minutes.

5. Stir in peppers, cover, and simmer for 5 minutes, leaving these vegetables crunchy.

Per Serving Calories: 251, Protein: 12 g, Carbohydrates: 44 g, Fiber: 14 g, Fat: 4.1 g, Saturated fat: 0.6 g, % of calories as fat: 14, Cholesterol: 0, Potassium: 718 mg, Sodium: 584 mg, Omega-3 fatty acids: 0.1 g

Exchanges Bread/starch: 2.2, Other carbs/sugar: 0, Very lean meat/protein: 0.2, Lean meat: 0, Fruit: 0, Vegetables: 1.1, Skim milk: 0, Fat: 0.7

CREAM OF BROCCOLI SOUP

I always want to order cream of broccoli soup in a restaurant, but know not to because of all the butter and cream that's usually used. I've been working for years to make a version that tastes just as good, without all the fat, and I think this is it. Be forewarned: This broccoli soup is chunky with all that great broccoli your body craves. [Serves 4]

2 tablespoons extra-virgin olive oil	2 teaspoons vegetable bouillon
3 cloves garlic	1 cup water
3 small onions, chopped	2 cups skim milk
One 2-pound bag frozen broccoli florets	8 ounces fat-free cream cheese
1 tablespoon yellow prepared mustard	2 ounces sharp cheddar cheese, shredded

Directions

1. Heat oil in a heavy pot over medium heat. Add garlic and onions, and sauté until onions are wilted. Do not brown garlic.

2. Add broccoli, mustard, bouillon, and water. Heat until broccoli is hot.

3. In a food processor, puree broccoli and onion mixture in batches with skim milk and cream cheese.

4. Return pureed mixture to pot and add cheddar cheese.

5. Heat until mixture is hot and cheese is melted.

Per Serving Calories: 323, Protein: 25 g, Carbohydrates: 30 g, Fiber: 8.4 g, Fat: 13.2 g, Saturated fat: 4.2 g, % of calories as fat: 35, Cholesterol: 22 mg, Potassium: 917 mg, Sodium: 846 mg, Omega-3 fatty acids: 0.3 g

Exchanges Bread/starch: 0.2, Other carbs/sugar: 0, Very lean meat/protein: 1.1, Lean meat: 0.5, Fruit: 0, Vegetables: 3.6, Skim milk: 0.5, Fat: 1.9

CHEESIEST POTATO SOUP

Simply said: awesomely delicious! [Serves 4]

1 tablespoon canola oil	2 cups water
3 garlic cloves, chopped	1 tablespoon vegetable bouillon
1 large white or Vidalia onion, chopped	2 cups skim milk
1 pound red potatoes	8 ounces 50% light cheddar cheese
3 celery stalks, chopped	Black pepper to taste

Directions

1. Heat oil in a heavy soup pot over medium heat.

2. Add garlic and onions, and sauté until onions are wilted. Remove from pan and set aside.

3. Scrub potatoes and dice with skin on. Place potatoes and celery in a pot with water and bouillon. Bring to a boil, lower heat, cover, and simmer until potatoes are fork-tender. Remove from heat.

4. Remove about three-fourths of potatoes and celery from pan. Place in a food processor in batches with onion-garlic mixture, skim milk, and puree. The pieces of red potato skin that do not puree will add color to the soup.

5. Return pureed mixture to the pot and add cheese and pepper.

6. Place pot back on burner over low heat and cook until cheese has melted, stirring occasionally.

Per Serving Calories: 316, Protein: 25 g, Carbohydrates: 33 g, Fiber: 3.4 g, Fat: 11.7 g, Saturated fat: 6.4 g, % of calories as fat: 31, Cholesterol: 32 mg, Potassium: 893 mg, Sodium: 850 mg, Omega-3 fatty acids: 0.32 g

Exchanges Bread/starch: 1, Other carbs/sugar: 0, Very lean meat/protein: 0, Lean meat: 2.2, Fruit: 0, Vegetables: 0.7, Skim milk: 0.5, Fat: 1.1

CREAM OF ASPARAGUS SOUP

Here's another easy soup that can be ready in minutes—and all year long—thanks to frozen asparagus. Besides an exceptionally satisfying bowl of soup, you're getting good fiber. [Serves 2]

1 tablespoon extra-virgin olive oil

3 cloves garlic, minced

1 cup chopped green onions

2 teaspoons vegetable bouillon

2 tablespoons water

One 10-ounce package frozen asparagus, thawed

¼ teaspoon black pepper, or to taste

6 ounces extra-firm tofu

2 cups soy milk or skim milk

Directions

1. Heat oil in a nonstick heavy kettle over low heat with garlic and onions. Sauté until onions are wilted. Do not burn garlic.

2. Add bouillon, water, asparagus, and pepper. Heat through.

3. Place the asparagus mixture in a food processor in batches with the tofu. Add just enough soy milk to make the creamy part of the soup smooth but still leave a few chunks of asparagus.

4. Return mixture to the pot, stir in remaining soy milk, and heat through.

Per Serving Calories: 305, Protein: 22 g, Carbohydrates: 26 g, Fiber: 3.3 g, Fat: 13.1 g, Saturated fat: 1.8 g, % of calories as fat: 38, Cholesterol: 0, Potassium: 909 mg, Sodium: 740 mg, Omega-3 fatty acids: 0.06 g

Exchanges Bread/starch: 1, Other carbs/sugar: 0, Very lean meat/protein: 0.9, Lean meat: 1.1, Fruit: 0, Vegetables: 1.8, Skim milk: 0, Fat: 1.6

THE BEST CHILI YOU'VE EVER HAD

This chili has become the highlight of nearly all parties we have in our home. Don't be daunted by the long list of ingredients. I've recreated that "chili seasoning in the packet" with my own list of seasonings—greatly slashing the sodium content. [Serves 8]

2 tablespoons canola oil

4 medium onions, chopped

3 cloves garlic, peeled and chopped

1 pound extra-lean ground beef

1 tablespoon very-low-sodium beef bouillon

8 celery stalks, cleaned and thinly sliced

4 cups water

One 30-ounce can kidney beans, drained and rinsed

One 29-ounce can no-salt-added crushed tomatoes

One 29-ounce can no-salt-added tomato puree

1 cup medium barley, uncooked

2 teaspoons granulated sugar

1 teaspoon ground basil

1 teaspoon ground oregano

3 tablespoons chili powder

¼ teaspoon black pepper

1 teaspoon salt

2 tablespoons ground cumin

1 can cooked black beans

1 medium green bell pepper, chopped

1 medium red bell pepper, chopped

1 medium yellow bell pepper, chopped

Directions

1. Heat oil in a large, heavy kettle over low heat. Add onions and garlic, and sauté 5 minutes to release flavors into oil.

2. Add ground beef, breaking it into crumbles, and bouillon. Increase heat and brown beef briefly.

3. Reduce heat to a simmer. Add celery, water, kidney beans, tomatoes, tomato puree, barley, sugar, basil, oregano, chili powder, pepper, cumin, and black beans. Stir well, cover, and simmer for 1 hour.

4. Stir in peppers and allow them to heat through, 2 to 3 minutes. The peppers will still be crisp-tender, adding a delightful crunch to the chili.

Per Serving Calories: 527, Protein: 32 g, Carbohydrates: 81 g, Fiber: 24.7 g, Fat: 10.6 g, Saturated fat: 2.6 g, % of calories as fat: 17, Cholesterol: 21 mg, Potassium: 1,901 mg, Sodium: 478 mg, Omega-3 fatty acids: 0.4 g

Exchanges Bread/starch: 3.2, Other carbs/sugar: 0.1, Very lean meat/protein: 0, Lean meat: 1.6, Fruit: 0, Vegetables: 5.3, Skim milk: 0, Fat: 0.8

SUN-DRIED TOMATO AND BLACK BEAN SOUP

Consider this one of your power soups—both in great nutrition and flavor. Your friends will think you've become a gourmet chef when you serve this soup, but it's so easy. As with all recipes that have beans, barley, and sun-dried tomatoes, you're getting lots of soluble fiber. [Serves 4]

2 tablespoons extra-virgin olive oil

2 large onions, chopped

2 cloves garlic, minced

⅓ cup black beans, uncooked

⅓ cup medium barley, uncooked

4 cups water

1 tablespoon vegetable bouillon

1 teaspoon cumin

3 cups sun-dried tomatoes

½ cup red wine

Two 10-ounce packages frozen Swiss chard

Directions

1. In a heavy soup kettle, heat oil with onions and garlic over low heat. Sauté gently about 5 minutes, or until onions have wilted.

2. Add black beans, barley, water, bouillon, cumin, tomatoes, and wine. Cover tightly and simmer for 45 minutes.

3. Add Swiss chard and simmer 15 to 20 minutes more, until chard has heated through.

Per Serving Calories: 359, Protein: 15 g, Carbohydrates: 58 g, Fiber: 13.5 g, Fat: 8.9 g, Saturated fat: 1.2 g, % of calories as fat: 20, Cholesterol: 0, Potassium: 2,337 mg, Sodium: 628 mg, Omega-3 fatty acids: 0.1 g

Exchanges Bread/starch: 1.4, Other carbs/sugar: 0, Very lean meat/protein: 0, Lean meat: 0, Fruit: 0, Vegetables: 6.3, Skim milk: 0, Fat: 1.8

WHITEFISH CHOWDER

I had forgotten some cod in the back of the freezer, so I wanted to find a way to cook it that would cover up how dry it had become. This recipe not only fit the bill but has become my favorite fish recipe. It's interestingly rich in flavor and a feast in itself. Chowder stores well in the refrigerator for about five days if tightly covered. [Serves 4]

2 tablespoons extra-virgin olive oil

1 medium yellow onion, chopped

3 cloves garlic, minced

2 cups celery, chopped

1 pound potatoes, scrubbed and cut into small chunks with skin on

4 carrots, peeled and sliced

1 pound cod or other whitefish such as haddock

1 tablespoon 33% reduced-sodium beef bouillon

1 tablespoon very-low-sodium beef bouillon

1 tablespoon crushed thyme

½ teaspoon black pepper

2 teaspoons garlic powder

1 cup fat-free sour cream

1 cup skim milk

5 tablespoons all-purpose flour

1 cup chopped fresh parsley

2 tablespoons lemon juice

Directions

1. Heat oil in a large nonstick kettle over low heat with onion and garlic. Sauté 5 minutes to release flavors into oil.

2. Add celery, potatoes, carrots, fish, both types of bouillon, thyme, pepper, and garlic powder. Add 2 to 3 cups water, just enough to cover vegetables and fish. Stir well (it's okay if fish breaks up), cover, and simmer for 30 to 40 minutes, until all vegetables are fork-tender.

3. Add sour cream and stir well to blend.

4. In a small bowl, mix milk with flour to make a smooth, lump-free paste. Add paste to chowder, stirring for 3 to 5 minutes, until mixture thickens.

5. Stir in fresh parsley and lemon juice.

Per Serving Calories: 422, Protein: 32 g, Carbohydrates: 57 g, Fiber: 7.3 g, Fat: 8.9 g, Saturated fat: 1.7 g, % of calories as fat: 18, Cholesterol: 56 mg, Potassium: 1,897 mg, Sodium: 917 mg, Omega-3 fatty acids: 0.3 g

Exchanges Bread/starch: 1.5, Other carbs/sugar: 0, Very lean meat/protein: 2.8, Lean meat: 0, Fruit: 0, Vegetables: 2.5, Skim milk: 0.8, Fat: 1.5

CHEDDAR CHEESE POTATO LEEK SOUP

A potato soup so rich in flavor you won't believe it's a healthy version. The combination of garlic and leeks sautéed slowly lends that richness, as does the pureed carrots with the potato. [Serves 4]

1 pound potatoes, scrubbed with peel on
4 carrots, peeled
1 tablespoon canola oil
1 clove garlic, peeled and minced
2 leeks, cleaned and sliced thinly

½ teaspoon salt
Black pepper to taste
2 cups skim milk
4 ounces 50% reduced-fat sharp cheddar cheese, grated

Directions

1. Cut potatoes into small pieces and slice carrots thinly.

2. Heat oil over low heat in medium-size kettle.

3. Add garlic and leeks, sautéing until wilted but not browned.

4. Add potatoes, carrots, salt, and pepper and enough water to cover mixture.

5. Cover and simmer until potatoes and carrots are fork-tender.

6. Drain vegetables.

7. Process vegetables with milk in small batches in food processor, until mostly smooth (a few chunks will remain).

8. Return to pot with cheese; heat until cheese is melted and soup is hot.

Per Serving Calories: 339, Protein: 18 g, Carbohydrates: 49 g, Fiber: 5.5 g, Fat: 9 g, Saturated fat: 3.9 g, % of calories as fat: 24, Cholesterol: 22 mg, Potassium: 1,057 mg, Sodium: 634 mg, Omega-3 fatty acids: 0.4 g

Exchanges Bread/starch: 1.7, Lean meat: 1.3, Vegetables: 2.6, Skim milk: 0.5, Fat: 0.9

Salads

GOAT CHEESE AND BRAZIL NUT SALAD

You'll love this heart- and waist-friendly way to use goat cheese, a wonderful but high-fat food. The secret is in mixing it with a like-textured food, fat-free cottage cheese. [Serves 2]

1 tablespoon balsamic vinegar
1 tablespoon extra-virgin olive oil
1 tablespoon Dijon mustard
1 teaspoon honey
Herbs de Provence to taste
4 cups chopped or torn romaine lettuce

1 red bell pepper, chopped
1 yellow bell pepper, chopped
½ cup fat-free extra-calcium cottage cheese
2 ounces goat cheese, crumbled (½ cup)
8 large Brazil nuts, sliced or chopped
¼ cup fat-free croutons

Directions

1. In a small bowl or cup, blend vinegar, oil, mustard, and honey. Add herbs. Set aside.

2. In a salad bowl, mix together the lettuce and bell peppers.

3. Place cottage cheese and goat cheese on top.

4. Sprinkle with Brazil nuts and croutons.

5. Drizzle with salad dressing and toss.

Per Serving Calories: 418, Protein: 19.7 g, Carbohydrates: 23.6 g, Fiber: 5.5 g, Fat: 29.4 g, Saturated fat: 10 g, % of calories as fat: 60, Cholesterol: 27 mg, Potassium: 780 mg, Sodium: 595 mg, Omega-3 fatty acids: 0.16 g

Exchanges Bread/starch: 0.2, Other carbs/sugar: 0.4, Very lean meat/protein: 1, Lean meat: 1.2, Fruit: 0, Vegetables: 2.1, Skim milk: 0, Fat: 5.1

SOUTHWEST SALAD

This salad is a great example of how mixing together a few unusual ingredients helps make healthier food interesting and satisfying. Millet provides the crunch as well as the whole grain goodness your body needs. If you have frozen millet, you can defrost it by placing it in a sieve and pouring boiling water over it. Hint: Hot bulgur, brown rice, or quinoa can be used instead of millet. [Serves 1]

2 cups romaine lettuce

2 cups arugula

½ cup cooked black beans (canned is okay, but rinse)

½ cup frozen corn, thawed

¼ chopped red onion

8 cherry tomatoes, halved

2 slices soy cheese, broken up

2 teaspoons extra-virgin olive oil

2 teaspoons balsamic vinegar

⅛ teaspoon chili powder

½ teaspoon granulated sugar

¼ cup hot cooked millet

Directions

1. Wash, dry, and chop or tear lettuce and arugula. Place in the bottom of individual salad bowl or plate.

2. Top with black beans, corn, onion, tomatoes, and cheese.

3. In a small bowl, whisk together oil, vinegar, chili powder, and sugar.

4. Put hot millet in bowl with sauce and toss.

5. Top salad with saucy millet and toss.

Per Serving Calories: 504, Protein: 25 g, Carbohydrates: 71 g, Fiber: 15.7 g, Fat: 16.1 g, Saturated fat: 1.7 g, % of calories as fat: 27, Cholesterol: 0, Potassium: 1,516 mg, Sodium: 521 mg, Omega-3 fatty acids: 0.4 g

Exchanges Bread/starch: 3.2, Other carbs/sugar: 0.2, Very lean meat/protein: 0.1, Lean meat: 0, Fruit: 0, Vegetables: 3.1, Skim milk: 0, Fat: 1.8

ZESTY THREE-BEAN SALAD

This salad dressing is versatile and scrumptious, and great to have on hand. As always, measure carefully. Toss together the salad ingredients with canned beans or cooked ones from your freezer. [Salad serves 1, but multiply as necesary; dressing serves 6, 1 tablespoon each]

Dressing

¼ cup extra-virgin olive oil

⅛ cup balsamic vinegar

½ clove garlic, minced

1 teaspoon Dijon mustard

⅛ teaspoon black pepper

¼ teaspoon salt

2 teaspoons dried basil

Salad (Makes enough for one person, but multiply as necessary)

¼ cup cooked white kidney beans (cannellini beans), canned is okay

¼ cup cooked black beans (canned is okay)

¼ cup cooked red kidney beans (canned is okay)

¼ of a 7-ounce jar roasted red peppers (in brine), chopped

½ medium tomato, chopped

2 cups chopped romaine lettuce

Directions

1. Whisk together the dressing ingredients until blended. Place in a tightly covered container and store in the refrigerator.

2. In a small bowl, toss together the 3 beans, red peppers, and tomato. Add 1 tablespoon dressing (mix well just before measuring) and toss gently.

3. Place bean mixture on lettuce.

Per Serving Calories: 305, Protein: 13 g, Carbohydrates: 43 g, Fiber: 10.6 g, Fat: 10.4 g, Saturated fat: 1.4 g, % of calories as fat: 29, Cholesterol: 0, Potassium: 817 mg, Sodium: 234 mg, Omega-3 fatty acids: 0.2 g

Exchanges Bread/starch: 1.9, Other carbs/sugar: 0.1, Very lean meat/protein: 0, Lean meat: 0, Fruit: 0, Vegetables: 1.8, Skim milk: 0, Fat: 1.9

FRESH VEGETABLE AND LENTIL SALAD

This salad is at once interesting and easy. The flavor bursts into a symphony with the blend of greens, lentils, and bulgur. It's so moist that it doesn't even need a dressing. If you would like one, just drizzle with your favorite vinegar and freshly ground black pepper. [Serves 1]

3 cups spinach

1 cup arugula

½ cup cooked lentils

½ cup cooked bulgur

1 cup sliced mushrooms

1 carrot, grated

1 cucumber, washed, sliced, and slices quartered with peel on

10 cherry tomatoes, halved

2 tablespoons walnut pieces

Directions

1. Wash, dry, and chop spinach and arugula. Place in an individual-serve salad bowl.

2. Top with lentils, bulgur, and mushrooms.

3. Add carrot, cucumber triangles, and cherry tomatoes.

4. Sprinkle with walnuts and toss.

Per Serving Calories: 410, Protein: 23 g, Carbohydrates: 63 g, Fiber: 21.2 g, Fat: 12 g, Saturated fat: 1.3 g, % of calories as fat: 24, Cholesterol: 0, Potassium: 2,129 mg, Sodium: 124 mg, Omega-3 fatty acids: 1.6 g

Exchanges Bread/starch: 2.4, Other carbs/sugar: 0, Very lean meat/protein: 0.2, Lean meat: 0.3, Fruit: 0, Vegetables: 4.9, Skim milk: 0, Fat: 1.6

QUINOA SALAD

This recipe uses one of my favorite secrets to gourmet and (don't tell anyone) healthy cooking: the use of tea bags while cooking the quinoa. (Note: Use flavored tea bags when cooking any grain to add a flavor explosion.) The combination of quinoa with greens and ordinary vegetables is exquisite! Green soybeans are also called edamame. They can be found in the freezer section with or without the pods. Buy without! [Serves 1]

¼ cup uncooked quinoa

2 spicy orange tea bags

⅔ cup water

3 cups spinach

1 cup watercress

10 cherry tomatoes, halved

1 cup sliced mushrooms

1 carrot, grated

½ cup cooked green soybeans, drained and cooled with ice cubes

1 to 2 tablespoons balsamic vinegar

Freshly ground black pepper to taste

Directions

1. Place quinoa and tea bags in a pot with ⅔ cup water. Bring to a boil, lower to a simmer, cover, and cook for 15 minutes.

2. Meanwhile, prepare salad by washing, drying, and chopping and tearing greens. Place in individual-serve salad bowl or on a salad plate.

3. In a small bowl, blend tomatoes, mushrooms, carrot, soybeans, and cooked quinoa; add vinegar and pepper. Toss.

4. Place quinoa mixture on top of greens.

Per Serving Calories: 393, Protein: 25 g, Carbohydrates: 60 g, Fiber: 13.8 g, Fat: 9.6 g, Saturated fat: 1.1 g, % of calories as fat: 20, Cholesterol: 0, Potassium: 2,324 mg, Sodium: 145 mg, Omega-3 fatty acids: 0.5 g

Exchanges Bread/starch: 2, Other carbs/sugar: 0, Very lean meat/protein: 1.4, Lean meat: 0, Fruit: 0, Vegetables: 6.2, Skim milk: 0, Fat: 0.9

MANDARIN BULGUR SALAD

Here's another great but easy salad that doesn't require dressing because it is already moist and bursting with flavor in its own right. [Serves 1]

3 cups romaine lettuce
½ cup cooked bulgur
¼ cup chopped red onion
½ cup chickpeas (also called garbanzo beans), cooked (canned is okay, but rinse and drain)
½ cup canned mandarin oranges, in juice, drained
6 to 8 (about 4 ounces) large strawberries, sliced, or 1 cup frozen strawberries, thawed
2 tablespoons chopped walnuts or walnut pieces

Directions

1. Wash, dry, and chop lettuce. Place in individual-serve salad bowl or on a salad plate.

2. Top with bulgur, onion, and chickpeas.

3. Arrange mandarin oranges and sliced strawberries on top.

4. Sprinkle with walnuts.

Per Serving Calories: 425, Protein: 17 g, Carbohydrates: 67 g, Fiber: 16.8 g, Fat: 12.8 g, Saturated fat: 1.3 g, % of calories as fat: 26, Cholesterol: 0, Potassium: 1,054 mg, Sodium: 26 mg, Omega-3 fatty acids: 1.6 g

Exchanges Bread/starch: 2.6, Other carbs/sugar: 0, Very lean meat/protein: 0.4, Lean meat: 0.3, Fruit: 1.2, Vegetables: 1.5, Skim milk: 0, Fat: 1.6

CHICKEN CAESAR SALAD

Adding canned/jarred artichoke hearts to this chicken Caesar salad pumps up the flavor—as well as the fiber and nutrients. For an extra zip, look for fat-free Caesar-flavored croutons. [Serves 1]

2 ounces cooked chicken breast (boneless, skinless), chopped

2 tablespoons grated Parmesan cheese

2 tablespoons fat-free Caesar dressing

1 cup cooked (or canned) artichoke hearts, chopped

3 cups romaine lettuce, chopped

½ cup fat-free seasoned croutons

Directions

1. In a small bowl, mix together chicken, Parmesan cheese, Caesar dressing, and artichoke hearts.

2. Place romaine lettuce on a salad plate and top with chicken-artichoke mixture.

3. Sprinkle with croutons.

Per Serving Calories: 392, Protein: 33 g, Carbohydrates: 46 g, Fiber: 13 g, Fat: 10 g, Saturated fat: 4 g, % of calories as fat: 23, Cholesterol: 56 mg, Potassium: 1,279 mg, Sodium: 1,440 mg, Omega-3 fatty acids: 0.3 g

Exchanges Bread/starch: 0.8, Other carbs: 1, Very lean meat/protein: 2.3, Lean meat: 0.7, Vegetables: 4.2, Fat: 1

SPINACH AND BARLEY SALAD

Whoever thought barley could taste this good? All mixed up with wonderful greens and sweet, fresh veggies—and topped with a rich olive oil dressing. You'll feel as though you're in a gourmet restaurant. [Serves 1]

3 cups spinach

1 cup arugula

¼ cup cooked barley

¼ cup kidney beans or adzuki beans

1 cup fresh or frozen broccoli florets

1 carrot, grated

1 stalk celery, chopped

10 cherry tomatoes, halved

1 tablespoon extra-virgin olive oil

1 tablespoon balsamic vinegar

1 clove garlic, minced

Freshly ground black pepper to taste

Directions

1. Wash, dry, and chop spinach and arugula. Place in a salad bowl or on a salad plate.

2. Top with barley, beans, broccoli, carrot, celery, and tomatoes.

3. Blend together the oil, vinegar, garlic, and pepper. Drizzle over the salad; toss.

Per Serving Calories: 384, Protein: 14 g, Carbohydrates: 55 g, Fiber: 17 g, Fat: 15.6 g, Saturated fat: 2.2 g, % of calories as fat: 34, Cholesterol: 0, Potassium: 1,909 mg, Sodium: 191 mg, Omega-3 fatty acids: 0.3 g

Exchanges Bread/starch: 1.8, Other carbs/sugar: 0.1, Very lean meat/protein: 0, Lean meat: 0, Fruit: 0, Vegetables: 4.6, Skim milk: 0, Fat: 2.6

FOUR-BEAN ITALIANO SALAD

Many of us love Italian salad at picnics and cookouts. Here's one you can serve as the main course. Just add fruit and milk for a complete meal. If you are serving as a main course, have a double portion. [Serves 4]

1 cup frozen green beans, thawed

½ cup canned wax beans, drained and rinsed

½ cup kidney beans (canned is okay, just rinse)

½ cup chickpeas (canned is okay, just rinse)

1 cup chopped red onion

2 tablespoons apple cider vinegar

1 tablespoon extra-virgin olive oil

1 tablespoon Mrs. Dash Classic Italiano or Italian seasoning

2 teaspoons granulated sugar

¼ teaspoon salt

Directions

1. In a medium-size bowl, combine green beans, wax beans, kidney beans, chickpeas, and onion.

2. In a small bowl, whisk together vinegar, oil, Mrs. Dash seasoning, sugar, and salt. Pour over salad and toss.

Per Serving Calories: 113, Protein: 4 g, Carbohydrates: 16 g, Fiber: 3.8 g, Fat: 4.2 g, Saturated fat: 0.6 g, % of calories as fat: 32, Cholesterol: 0, Potassium: 218 mg, Sodium: 303 mg, Omega-3 fatty acids: 0.1 g

Exchanges Bread/starch: 0.6, Other carbs/sugar: 0.1, Very lean meat/protein: 0.3, Lean meat: 0, Fruit: 0, Vegetables: 0.6, Skim milk: 0, Fat: 0.7

Fish

LEMON PEPPER SIZZLED TILAPIA

Tilapia is a wonderful mild yet firm fish that comes from the rain forests of South America. If you cannot find tilapia, substitute orange roughy, cod, or snapper. Mixing olive oil and lemon juice is a wonderful trick I use to cut the fat that the fish absorbs, and it bumps up the flavor considerably. [Serves 2]

2 tablespoons fresh lemon juice
1 tablespoon extra-virgin olive oil
10 ounces tilapia
1 teaspoon Mrs. Dash Lemon Pepper or any brand without sodium

Directions

1. Place lemon juice and oil in large nonstick skillet over medium-high heat.

2. Place tilapia in skillet and sprinkle with lemon pepper.

3. Cook each side for 4 to 6 minutes, until fish is cooked through.

Per Serving Calories: 271, Protein: 36 g, Carbohydrates: 1 g, Fiber: 0.1 g, Fat: 12.4 g, Saturated fat: 2.3 g, % of calories as fat: 42, Cholesterol: 108 mg, Potassium: 695 mg, Sodium: 109 mg, Omega-3 fatty acids: 1.2 g

Exchanges Bread/starch: 0, Other carbs/sugar: 0, Very lean meat/protein: 5.2, Lean meat: 0, Fruit: 0.1, Vegetables: 0, Skim milk: 0, Fat: 1.9

GARLIC-SAUTÉED FLOUNDER AND VEGETABLE RIBBONS

This fantastically beautiful meal is ready in minutes. Don't hesitate to serve it to company! [Serves 4]

4 carrots, peeled

2 small green zucchini, with peel on and washed

1 tablespoon extra-virgin olive oil

2 cloves garlic, minced

2 teaspoons vegetable bouillon

2 to 4 tablespoons water

1 pound flounder

Directions

1. After peeling carrots use the peeler and create long carrot ribbons, work the carrot all the way down to the white portion.

2. Peel long green ribbons from the skin of the zucchini, working down to the white portion (use the inner parts of the carrots and zucchini for making soup).

3. Heat oil in a large nonstick skillet over low heat. Add garlic and sauté for 3 to 5 minutes to release flavor into oil.

4. Add bouillon and 2 tablespoons water. Increase heat to medium-high and add vegetable ribbons. Sauté for 5 minutes. Add additional water if more cooking liquid is needed.

5. Remove vegetable ribbons from pan and place flounder in middle of pan. Cook each side for 3 to 5 minutes, depending on thickness.

6. Place vegetable strips on top of fish, cover, and turn heat off. Allow just enough time to reheat cooked vegetable strips.

Per Serving Calories: 214, Protein: 31 g, Carbohydrates: 10 g, Fiber: 2.3 g, Fat: 5.7 g, Saturated fat: 1.2 g, % of calories as fat: 24, Cholesterol: 81 mg, Potassium: 847 mg, Sodium: 440 mg, Omega-3 fatty acids: 0.1 g

Exchanges Bread/starch: 0, Other carbs/sugar: 0, Very lean meat/protein: 3.9, Lean meat: 0, Fruit: 0, Vegetables: 1.5, Skim milk: 0, Fat: 0.7

SOUTHWEST TUNA AND SALSA

You're creating your own fresh salsa in this great and easy recipe! [Serves 4]

Vegetable oil spray
¼ cup fresh lime juice
1 tablespoon chili powder
¾ teaspoon ground cumin
1 tablespoon granulated sugar
½ cup chopped fresh cilantro or
   1 tablespoon dried

1 cup chopped green onions (about 4)
1 large red bell pepper, cored and finely chopped
1 large green bell pepper, cored and finely chopped
1 large yellow bell pepper, cored and finely
   chopped
2 large tomatoes, chopped
1 pound tuna fillet, cut into 4 equal portions

Directions

1. Heat oven to 400 degrees F. Coat a 9 × 12 baking pan with vegetable oil spray.

2. In a medium-size bowl, whisk together lime juice, chili powder, cumin, sugar, and cilantro.

3. Stir in onions, peppers, and tomatoes.

4. Place tuna fillets in baking pan. Pour salsa mixture on top.

5. Cover tightly and bake for 15 to 20 minutes, or until tuna flakes. Some vegetables will still be crisp-tender.

Per Serving Calories: 230, Protein: 35 g, Carbohydrates: 18 g, Fiber: 4.1 g, Fat: 2.5 g, Saturated fat: 0.6 g, % of calories as fat: 10, Cholesterol: 68 mg, Potassium: 1,214 mg, Sodium: 93 mg, Omega-3 fatty acids: 0.4 g

Exchanges Bread/starch: 0, Other carbs/sugar: 0.2, Very lean meat/protein: 4.4, Lean meat: 0, Fruit: 0.1, Vegetables: 2.6, Skim milk: 0, Fat: 0

SWEET-AND-SOUR TUNA

This version of tuna, so great tasting and so wonderfully high in omega-3 fats, might be served with rice. Try out your new interest in grains and serve over millet, quinoa, or bulgur. You'll love the great topping to your grain base. [Serves 2]

1 tablespoon canola oil

½ cup chopped red onion

10 ounces tuna fillet

1 red bell pepper, cored and cut into slices

1 green bell pepper, cored and cut into slices

1 carrot, peeled and very thinly sliced

2 tablespoons distilled vinegar

1 teaspoon black pepper or less to taste

1 tablespoon cornstarch

½ cup orange juice

½ cup canned crushed pineapple

Directions

1. Heat oil in a large nonstick skillet over medium heat. Add onion and sauté for 5 minutes to release flavor into oil.

2. Increase heat to high and add tuna. Brown each side for 3 minutes. Lower heat and add bell peppers, carrot, vinegar, and pepper. Cover and simmer for 5 minutes. Vegetables will still be crisp-tender.

3. Blend cornstarch into orange juice. Add to pan, stirring until mixture thickens.

4. Stir in crushed pineapple.

Per Serving Calories: 376, Protein: 43 g, Carbohydrates: 30 g, Fiber: 4.6 g, Fat: 9 g, Saturated fat: 1.1 g, % of calories as fat: 22, Cholesterol: 85 mg, Potassium: 1,271 mg, Sodium: 67 mg, Omega-3 fatty acids: 1.1 g

Exchanges Bread/starch: 0.3, Other carbs/sugar: 0, Very lean meat/protein: 5.4, Lean meat: 0, Fruit: 0.9, Vegetables: 2.3, Skim milk: 0, Fat: 1.3

PINEAPPLE SALMON

You can prepare this wonderful salmon dish in just minutes, leaving you time for exercise while you wait for it to bake. [Serves 4]

1 pound salmon fillet
1 medium green pepper
One 8.25-ounce can pineapple rings (in juice)
½ cup chopped green onion
Black pepper to taste

Directions

1. Preheat oven to 425 degrees F. Line a 9 × 12 baking dish with aluminum foil, using enough to wrap the salmon tightly.

2. Place salmon fillet, skin side down, on foil.

3. Arrange pineapple rings on top of salmon and pour juice on top.

4. Sprinkle with green onion and pepper.

5. Seal foil tightly and place pan in oven. Bake for 20 to 30 minutes, depending on thickness of salmon. It will flake when done.

Per Serving Calories: 172, Protein: 22 g, Carbohydrates: 12 g, Fiber: 1.5 g, Fat: 3.8 g, Saturated fat: 0.6 g, % of calories as fat: 20, Cholesterol: 56 mg, Potassium: 502 mg, Sodium: 75 mg, Omega-3 fatty acids: 1.1 g

Exchanges Bread/starch: 0, Other carbs/sugar: 0, Very lean meat/protein: 3.1, Lean meat: 0, Fruit: 0.6, Vegetables: 0.6, Skim milk: 0, Fat: 0.4

FOILED SALMON AND VEGGIES

I believe that you can never have too many ways to cook salmon. This is another of my easy "pack up and bake" recipes. I've made it incredibly easy by using frozen veggies. Next time you see a great deal on salmon, freeze it in 4-ounce portions, and then you'll be ready to make a nearly complete meal like this. When you pull out the salmon, just pull out one of your cooked grain portions to accompany this deliciously different, yet so easy, recipe. [Serves 2]

One 8- to 10-ounce salmon fillet

1 teaspoon extra-virgin olive oil

Freshly ground black pepper to taste

¼ to ½ teaspoon ground ginger

One 10-ounce box frozen cauliflower

One 10-ounce box frozen carrots

One 7.25-ounce jar roasted red peppers (in brine, not oil), drained

Directions

1. Preheat oven to 425 degrees F. Line a 9 × 12 baking dish with aluminum foil, using enough to wrap the salmon tightly.

2. Place salmon fillet, skin side down, on foil.

3. Rub oil into salmon.

4. Sprinkle with pepper and ginger.

5. Top with cauliflower, carrots, and red peppers.

6. Wrap foil tightly around salmon and vegetables. Bake for 20 to 30 minutes, or until salmon flakes.

Per Serving Calories: 352, Protein: 34.7 g, Carbohydrates: 25.4 g, Fiber: 8.6 g, Fat: 12.8 g, Saturated fat: 2 g, % of calories as fat: 32, Cholesterol: 80.5 mg, Potassium: 1,247 mg, Sodium: 250 mg, Omega-3 fatty acids: 2.69 g

Exchanges Bread/starch: 0, Other carbs/sugar: 0, Very lean meat/protein: 4.1, Lean meat: 0, Fruit: 0, Vegetables: 4.9, Skim milk: 0, Fat: 2

LEMON-FRESH SALMON LOAF

The fresh taste of lemon and the richness of the oat bran bread join together to create a wonderfully rich, yet gentle, comfort food. The leftovers are great cold as sandwiches or just as an easy lunch. [Serves 4]

Vegetable oil spray

15 ounces canned pink salmon, drained and with bone and skin removed

4 egg whites or ½ cup liquid egg white substitute

4 slices oat bran bread, broken into tiny pieces

½ red onion, minced

¼ cup lemon juice

¼ teaspoon black pepper

Directions

1. Preheat oven to 350 degrees F. Coat a large loaf pan with vegetable oil spray.

2. Place all ingredients in a bowl and blend together with a fork. Alternatively, place all ingredients in a food processor and pulse until blended.

3. Place mixture in a loaf pan and pat down.

4. Bake for 40 minutes.

Per Serving Calories: 258, Protein: 31 g, Carbohydrates: 15 g, Fiber: 1.7 g, Fat: 7.8 g, Saturated fat: 1.9 g, % of calories as fat: 28, Cholesterol: 58 mg, Potassium: 515 mg, Sodium: 814 mg, Omega-3 fatty acids: 1.85 g

Exchanges Bread/starch: 0.8, Other carbs/sugar: 0, Very lean meat/protein: 3.9, Lean meat: 0, Fruit: 0.1, Vegetables: 0.3, Skim milk: 0, Fat: 1.1

GINGER-SEARED SALMON AND SWISS CHARD

Mediterranean cooking wouldn't be complete without fish, nor would heart-healthy menus. Salmon is rich in omega-3 fatty acids. Tuna, mackerel, and trout are other great sources. This recipe also includes goodly amounts of a fabulous vegetable, Swiss chard, and gives you an easy way to include it in your eating plan. You'll see that one pound cooks down to a few bites per person. [Serves 4]

1 tablespoon dark sesame oil

¼ cup finely chopped fresh ginger (after peeling)

Four 4-ounce pieces salmon fillet

1 pound red Swiss chard, julienned

1 cup finely chopped green onions, tops and bottoms

½ cup finely chopped fresh cilantro leaves

3 tablespoons reduced-sodium soy sauce

1 cup grated carrot

Directions

1. In a large, deep nonstick skillet, heat oil and ginger over high heat. Add salmon and sear each side for 2 minutes.

2. Lower heat to medium. Remove salmon from pan, place Swiss chard in bottom of pan, and top with salmon pieces. Add onions and cilantro.

3. Sprinkle soy sauce on top.

4. Cover tightly and simmer for 15–20 minutes, until fish flakes and Swiss chard wilts. The Swiss chard quickly creates more cooking liquid. Baste twice during cooking, covering tightly afterward.

5. Divide vegetables and fish among 4 plates. Garnish each with ¼ cup grated carrot.

Per Serving Calories: 218, Protein: 26 g, Carbohydrates: 11 g, Fiber: 3.9 g, Fat: 7.9 g, Saturated fat: 1.6 g, % of calories as fat: 33, Cholesterol: 53 mg, Potassium: 1,064 mg, Sodium: 713 mg, Omega-3 fatty acids: 1.1 g

Exchanges Bread/starch: 0, Other carbs/sugar: 0, Very lean meat/protein: 3.3, Lean meat: 0, Fruit: 0, Vegetables: 2, Skim milk: 0, Fat: 1.1

CRAB À LA TUNA CAKES

Ah, crab cakes—often a fabulous beginning to a fine meal. This version uses canned tuna simply to squeeze more omega-3 fats into your menu and also because it is inexpensive. Feel free to make this in larger patties for a whole meal. This recipe uses another low-fat cooking secret: mixing lemon juice and fat for "frying." It greatly cuts the calories but still allows the product to brown. This works particularly well with fish. [Serves 6]

4 egg whites, lightly beaten, or ⅓ cup liquid egg white substitute

5 tablespoons lemon juice (divided)

½ teaspoon black pepper

1 teaspoon extra-hot horseradish

⅓ cup fat-free mayonnaise

2 slices whole grain bread (preferably an especially hearty one), torn into small chunks

One 6-ounce can albacore tuna, drained

¼ cup minced green onion

¼ cup minced yellow pepper

¼ cup minced red pepper

¼ cup minced cilantro

1 tablespoon canola oil

Directions

1. In a small mixing bowl, stir together the egg whites, 4 tablespoons lemon juice, pepper, horseradish, and mayonnaise.

2. Add bread and use a fork to blend well.

3. Add tuna and use a fork again to blend.

4. Fold in onion, peppers, and cilantro. Divide mixture into 12 equal portions and form into cakes.

5. Heat oil and remaining 1 tablespoon lemon juice in a nonstick skillet over high heat. Add tuna cakes and cook 2–4 minutes per side, or until browned.

Per Serving Calories: 101, Protein: 10 g, Carbohydrates: 9 g, Fiber: 1.4 g, Fat: 3.5 g, Saturated fat: 0.7 g, % of calories as fat: 30, Cholesterol: 13 mg, Potassium: 178 mg, Sodium: 286 mg, Omega-3 fatty acids: 0.3 g

Exchanges Bread/starch: 0.2, Other carbs/sugar: 0.2, Very lean meat/protein: 1.4, Lean meat: 0, Fruit: 0.1, Vegetables: 0.3, Skim milk: 0, Fat: 0.5

LEMON-AND-ORANGE-ROASTED RED SNAPPER

So simple and yet so elegant. (The best part: So easy.) [Serves 4]

Vegetable oil spray
1 pound red snapper
2 teaspoons extra-virgin olive oil
½ to 1 teaspoon Mrs. Dash Lemon Pepper
1 medium orange

Directions

1. Preheat oven to 400 degrees F. Line a baking pan with aluminum foil. Coat with vegetable oil spray.

2. Place snapper on foil, skin side down.

3. Rub oil into snapper. Sprinkle with lemon pepper.

4. Slice orange thinly with rind on and lay slices on top of snapper.

5. Seal foil tightly around snapper and bake for 15 to 20 minutes, depending on thickness of fish; it will flake when done.

6. Unseal foil and cut snapper into 4 portions. Place orange slice on top of each portion.

Per Serving Calories: 112, Protein: 16 g, Carbohydrates: 4 g, Fiber: 0.8 g, Fat: 3.3 g, Saturated fat: 0.5 g, % of calories as fat: 27, Cholesterol: 28 mg, Potassium: 370 mg, Sodium: 34 mg, Omega-3 fatty acids: 0.2 g

Exchanges Bread/starch: 0, Other carbs/sugar: 0, Very lean meat/protein: 2.1, Lean meat: 0, Fruit: 0.3, Vegetables: 0, Skim milk: 0, Fat: 0.4

"LOBSTER" WITH BASIL-CAPER DRIZZLE

The imitation shellfish products are excellent choices to have on hand for a quick gourmet meal, especially for those allergic to shellfish. Just watch portion size because sodium tends to be high. This wonderful meal is easy and yet great for company. [Serves 2]

Sauce

½ cup chopped fresh basil

1 tablespoon capers

1 tablespoon light mayonnaise

1 tablespoon country Dijon mustard

2 tablespoons white rice vinegar

⅛ teaspoon black pepper

1 tablespoon extra-virgin olive oil

Salad

4 arugula leaves

6 Bibb lettuce leaves

4 slices tomato

8 large asparagus spears, steamed and cut on the diagonal into 1-inch slices

8 ounces imitation lobster, sliced

Directions

1. Place all sauce ingredients in a small bowl and whisk until smooth.

2. Arrange arugula and lettuce leaves on 2 plates. Top with tomato slices, asparagus, and lobster slices.

3. Drizzle sauce on top.

Per Serving Calories: 261, Protein: 19 g, Carbohydrates: 22 g, Fiber: 3.5 g, Fat: 9.5 g, Saturated fat: 1.4 g, % of calories as fat: 34, Cholesterol: 58 mg, Potassium: 711 mg, Sodium: 450 mg, Omega-3 fatty acids: 0.1 g

Exchanges Bread/starch: 0.9, Other carbs/sugar: 0.1, Very lean meat/protein: 1.8, Lean meat: 0, Fruit: 0, Vegetables: 1.4, Skim milk: 0, Fat: 1.7

ROSEMARY-HORSERADISH–POTATO-ENCRUSTED CHILEAN SEA BASS

This recipe requires a little more work, but it's well worth it. Rosemary complements sea bass especially well. [Serves 4]

1 pound baking potatoes, scrubbed and cut into pieces with peel on

½ cup low-fat cream cheese

Vegetable oil spray

2 teaspoons horseradish, or to taste

2 tablespoons chopped fresh rosemary (preferably) or 2 teaspoons dried

4 egg whites or ⅓ cup liquid egg white substitute

1 pound sea bass, cut into 4 equal pieces

Directions

1. Boil potatoes until fork-tender. Drain and return to pot.

2. Add cream cheese and place over low heat for 5 minutes; potatoes mash better with hot cream cheese.

3. Preheat oven to 425 degrees F. Coat a baking sheet heavily with vegetable oil spray.

4. Turn heat off under potatoes. Add horseradish, rosemary, and egg whites. Mash with an electric mixer or by hand.

5. Divide potato mixture into 8 portions. Place 4 portions on cookie sheet far enough apart to allow for fish. Place fish fillet on top of each potato portion. Put another potato portion on top.

6. Using your fingers, mold the potatoes around the fish. Coat the top of each with vegetable oil spray.

7. Bake in the oven for 20 to 30 minutes, or until potatoes are crusty and just slightly browned.

Per Serving Calories: 326, Protein: 34 g, Carbohydrates: 26 g, Fiber: 2.5 g, Fat: 8.9 g, Saturated fat: 4.2 g, % of calories as fat: 25, Cholesterol: 77 mg, Potassium: 869 mg, Sodium: 231 mg, Omega-3 fatty acids: 1 g

Exchanges Bread/starch: 1.6, Other carbs/sugar: 0, Very lean meat/protein: 4.1, Lean meat: 0.4, Fruit: 0, Vegetables: 0, Skim milk: 0, Fat: 1

TOMATO-AND-HERB-ROASTED RED SNAPPER

Another easy yet fabulously different fish recipe. This fish is especially great served over a bed of spinach pasta that has been tossed with lemon juice and chopped steamed spinach. [Serves 2]

1 pound snapper	½ teaspoon salt
1 teaspoon extra-virgin olive oil	2 cloves garlic, minced
1 tablespoon lemon juice	2 tomatoes, chopped
1 teaspoon ground basil	¼ cup minced Italian leaf parsley for garnish
1 teaspoon oregano	

Directions

1. Preheat oven to 350 degrees F. Line a 9 × 12 baking pan with aluminum foil, using enough to wrap the snapper tightly.

2. Lay snapper fillet, skin side down, in the center of the foil.

3. Rub oil into snapper. Drizzle with lemon juice and sprinkle with basil, oregano, salt, and garlic. Place tomatoes on top.

4. Wrap foil tightly around snapper. Bake for 30 minutes.

5. Sprinkle each portion with 2 tablespoons parsley.

Per Serving Calories: 214, Protein: 33 g, Carbohydrates: 9 g, Fiber: 2.4 g, Fat: 5 g, Saturated fat: 0.9 g, % of calories as fat: 21, Cholesterol: 56 mg, Potassium: 971 mg, Sodium: 665 mg, Omega-3 fatty acids: 0.4 g

Exchanges Bread/starch: 0, Other carbs/sugar: 0, Very lean meat/protein: 4.3, Lean meat: 0, Fruit: 0, Vegetables: 1.3, Skim milk: 0, Fat: 0.5

GINGER-SEARED SOLE ON A BED OF GINGER-STEAMED LENTILS

A few simple ingredients create a wonderful feast. Feel free to substitute any fish.
[Serves 4]

2 cups uncooked lentils

3 tablespoons minced fresh ginger (divided)

6 cups water

1 tablespoon sesame oil

3 garlic cloves, minced

1 pound sole

½ cup minced cilantro

1 cup mandarin orange sections without juice

Directions

1. Place lentils, 1 tablespoon ginger, and water in a heavy saucepan over medium-high heat. Bring to a boil. Lower heat and simmer for 45 minutes, until lentils are fork-tender.

2. When lentils have simmered for 15 minutes, heat oil over low heat in a large non-stick skillet with remaining 2 tablespoons ginger and garlic. Sauté for 5 minutes to release flavor into oil.

3. Increase heat to medium-high and add sole. Sear each side for 2–3 minutes.

4. Reduce heat to medium-low. Sprinkle with cilantro, cover, and steam just until fish flakes.

5. When lentils are fork-tender, toss with orange sections.

6. Place one-fourth of lentil mixture on each plate and top with one-fourth of sole.

Per Serving Calories: 402, Protein: 42 g, Carbohydrates: 47 g, Fiber: 16.9 g, Fat: 5.8 g, Saturated fat: 1 g, % of calories as fat: 13, Cholesterol: 60 mg, Potassium: 1,228 mg, Sodium: 97 mg, Omega-3 fatty acids: 0.1 g

Exchanges Bread/starch: 2.6, Other carbs/sugar: 0, Very lean meat/protein: 3.6, Lean meat: 0, Fruit: 0.3, Vegetables: 0.1, Skim milk: 0, Fat: 0.7

SUN-DRIED TOMATO AND TUNA QUICHE

I love quiche but hate all the fat in the traditional crust. That is why I worked hard to create a crust that leaves lots of calories for other ingredients. Use this crust recipe for other quiches—just change the seasoning. [Serves 4]

Vegetable oil spray

2 cups cooked brown rice

1 tablespoon extra-virgin olive oil

1¼ cups liquid egg white substitute (divided)

2 tablespoons Mrs. Dash Classic Italiano or Italian seasoning (divided)

6 ounces tuna canned in water, drained

1 cup chopped green onions

2 cups chopped sun-dried tomatoes

2 tablespoons grated Parmesan cheese

1 cup skim milk

½ teaspoon salt

Directions

1. Heat oven to 350 degrees F. Coat a deep-dish pie plate with vegetable oil spray.

2. Combine rice, oil, ¼ cup egg whites, and 1 tablespoon Mrs. Dash seasoning in a bowl. Whisk together.

3. Press rice mixture into pie plate, forming a crust. Place in oven for 10 minutes.

4. Meanwhile, in a medium-size bowl, stir together remaining 1 tablespoon Mrs. Dash seasoning, tuna, green onions, tomatoes, cheese, remaining 1 cup egg whites, skim milk, and salt.

5. After crust has baked for 10 minutes, pour tuna mixture into crust.

6. Return to oven and bake for 35–40 minutes, or until a knife inserted in the middle comes out clean.

7. Let stand 10–15 minutes before cutting into 4 equal servings.

Per Serving Calories: 342, Protein: 29 g, Carbohydrates: 43 g, Fiber: 6.1 g, Fat: 6.6 g, Saturated fat: 1.6 g, % of calories as fat: 17, Cholesterol: 16 mg, Potassium: 1,351 mg, Sodium: 659 mg, Omega-3 fatty acids: 0.2 g

Exchanges Bread/starch: 1.4, Other carbs/sugar: 0, Very lean meat/protein: 2.5, Lean meat: 0.2, Fruit: 0, Vegetables: 3.2, Skim milk: 0.2, Fat: 0.8

Snacks/Desserts

BERRY FRESH CHEESECAKE

Has anyone ever told you that you absolutely had to eat a cheesecake for your good health? Well, I am! This cheesecake is loaded with calcium, which is great for your bones. While we've included nutrition information for cottage cheese that is not calcium fortified, do try to choose the calcium-fortified version to obtain even more calcium. The berry topping bumps up your fiber. Another secret to keeping the fat low: There isn't a crust. This saves precious calories and fat grams for better things. So enjoy this wonderful recipe for breakfast, dessert, or a healthy snack. A large food processor is recommended for this recipe because it allows you to dump in all the ingredients, zap, and bake. [Serves 8]

Cheesecake

Vegetable oil spray

One 8-ounce package low-fat cream cheese at room temperature

One 8-ounce package nonfat cream cheese at room temperature

1 pound nonfat cottage cheese

4 egg whites or ⅓ cup liquid egg white substitute

¼ cup brown Sugar Twin

½ cup granulated sugar

1 teaspoon lemon juice

1 tablespoon vanilla extract

3 tablespoons cornstarch

Sauce

2 cups frozen unsweetened mixed berries, thawed, or fresh or frozen raspberries or strawberries (choose those frozen without sugar)

Spritz of lemon juice (optional)

Directions

1. Preheat oven to 350 degrees F. Coat a deep-dish pie plate with vegetable oil spray.

2. In a large food processor, combine both packages of cream cheese, cottage cheese, and egg whites. Whirl until smooth.

3. Add brown Sugar Twin, sugar, 1 teaspoon lemon juice, vanilla, and cornstarch. Whirl again until mixture is smooth.

4. Pour into pie plate and level with a rubber spatula.

5. Bake for 25–35 minutes, or until a knife inserted in the middle comes out clean. (The cheesecake will puff up considerably while baking and then fall when you remove it from the oven. This is okay. The edges will become a slight golden brown but should not brown excessively.)

6. Remove from the oven and let cool on a rack briefly, then place in the refrigerator to chill.

7. Just before serving, place berries in a food processor and process until smooth. Add a spritz of lemon juice for a little zest if desired. Top cheesecake with fruit.

Per Serving Calories: 222, Protein: 16 g, Carbohydrates: 26 g, Fiber: 2.1 g, Fat: 5.6 g, Saturated fat: 3.4 g, % of calories as fat: 23, Cholesterol: 21 mg, Potassium: 262 mg, Sodium: 517 mg, Omega-3 fatty acids: 0.1 g

Exchanges Bread/starch: 0.4, Other carbs/sugar: 0.7, Very lean meat/protein: 1.7, Lean meat: 0.4, Fruit: 0.2, Vegetables: 0, Skim milk: 0, Fat: 0.9

GINGER-POACHED PEARS

We all get tired of plain old fruit, no matter how "good for us" it is. Try this easy recipe to break the monotony. Enjoy these pears as part of your breakfast, as a snack, or at a dinner party with a scoop of frozen vanilla yogurt. The extras store well in the refrigerator for up to four days. They are good hot or cold. [Serves 4]

1 cup water
4 green tea bags
One 1-inch piece of ginger, finely diced
2 teaspoons packed brown sugar
2 medium pears

Directions

1. Preheat oven to 350 degrees F. Coat a small oven-safe casserole with vegetable oil spray.

2. Place 1 cup water, tea bags, ginger, and sugar in the casserole and stir.

3. Cut pears into quarters and remove core, but leave skin on. Slice quarters one additional time. Place pear slices in cooking liquid. If pears are not entirely covered with liquid, add enough water to cover. You can also add more ginger and another tea bag.

4. Cover casserole and bake for 30 minutes, or until pears are fork-tender.

Per Serving (½ pear and ¼ of the cooking liquid) Calories: 58, Protein: 0.3 g, Carbohydrates: 15 g, Fiber: 2 g, Fat: 0.3 g, Saturated fat: 0, % of calories as fat: 5, Cholesterol: 0, Potassium: 114 mg, Sodium: 1 mg, Omega-3 fatty acids: 0

Exchanges Bread/starch: 0, Other carbs/sugar: 0.1, Very lean meat/protein: 0, Lean meat: 0, Fruit: 0.8, Vegetables: 0, Skim milk: 0, Fat: 0

GINGER SNAP APPLE

This recipe is a great way to "have your cake and eat it, too." I've combined the best of good nutrition with fabulous sweet flavor for a real treat. This is definitely "company good" but easy to make for yourself. With a glass of nonfat milk on the side or topped with yogurt, this dish makes a great breakfast, too. The leftovers refrigerate well up to four days. [Serves 4]

Vegetable oil spray

3 medium apples

2 tablespoons lemon juice

2 ounces walnuts, chopped

2 ounces ginger snap cookies (about 14), broken into small pieces

1 teaspoon packed brown sugar

2 teaspoons vanilla extract

One 1-inch piece of ginger, minced

½ cup water

Directions

1. Preheat oven to 350 degrees F. Coat 4 custard cups with vegetable oil spray.

2. Wash and quarter apples with peel. Cut into thin slices. Place in a medium bowl with lemon juice and toss.

3. In another small bowl, blend walnuts, cookies, brown sugar, vanilla, ginger, and water (it will become gooey).

4. Transfer mixture to bowl with apples and toss well to mix and coat apples.

5. Spoon apple mixture into custard cups.

6. Bake for 30 minutes.

Per Serving Calories: 221, Protein: 4 g, Carbohydrates: 31 g, Fiber: 3.8 g, Fat: 9.7 g, Saturated fat: 0.8 g, % of calories as fat: 37, Cholesterol: 0, Potassium: 278 mg, Sodium: 88 mg, Omega-3 fatty acids: 0.5 g

Exchanges Bread/starch: 0, Other carbs/sugar: 0.8, Very lean meat/protein: 0.4, Lean meat: 0, Fruit: 1.1, Vegetables: 0, Skim milk: 0, Fat: 1.8

RICH CHOCOLATE SHAKE

Chocolate lovers of the world: Here's a chocolate shake you can enjoy with reckless abandon. [Serves 1]

⅔ cup chocolate sorbet
½ cup low-fat vanilla yogurt
½ cup skim milk

Directions

Blend all in blender or food processor.

Per Serving Calories: 307, Protein: 13 g, Carbohydrates: 60 g, Fiber: 2.67 g, Fat: 1.7 g, Saturated fat: 1.1 g, % of calories as fat: 5, Cholesterol: 8.2 mg, Potassium: 471 mg, Sodium: 237 mg, Omega-3 fatty acids: 0

Exchanges Bread/starch: 0, Other carbs/sugar: 3.5, Very lean meat/protein: 0, Lean meat: 0, Fruit: 0, Vegetables: 0, Skim milk: 0.5, Fat: 0.4

DOUBLE RASPBERRY SHAKE

This shake is as nutritionally packed as it is refreshing and guiltfully delicious. Note the great fiber you get, in addition to loads of vitamins and potassium. [Serves 1]

½ cup raspberry sorbet
½ cup fresh or frozen raspberries
½ cup skim milk
3 tablespoons skim milk powder

Directions

Blend all in blender or food processor.

Per Serving Calories: 247, Protein: 10 g, Carbohydrates: 51 g, Fiber: 6 g, Fat: 0.6 g, Saturated fat: 0.2 g, % of calories as fat: 0, Cholesterol: 2 mg, Potassium: 605 mg, Sodium: 148 mg, Omega-3 fatty acids: 0

Exchanges Bread/starch: 0, Other carbs/sugar: 1.5, Very lean meat/protein: 0, Lean meat: 0, Fruit: 1.5, Vegetables: 0, Skim milk: 1.0, Fat: 0

FROZEN PEACH SHAKE

Pop just two ingredients in the blender for a refreshing snack! [Serves 1]

1 container of peach yogurt (about 80 to 100 calories)
½ cup low-fat frozen vanilla yogurt

Directions

Blend ingredients in blender until smooth.

Per Serving Calories: 195, Protein: 13.8 g, Carbohydrates: 33.1 g, Fiber: 0 g, Fat: 1.3 g, Saturated Fat: 0.8 g, % of calories as fat: 6, Cholesterol: 8.56 mg, Potassium: 543.4 mg, Sodium: 172.4 mg, Omega-3 fatty acids: 0 g

Exchanges Bread/starch: 0, Other carbs/sugar: 2.2, Very lean meat/protein: 0, Lean meat: 0, Fruit: 0, Vegetables: 0, Skim milk: 0, Fat: 0.3

LEMON TORTE

Here's another magical dessert recipe that is also great for you. And you can have it for breakfast, too. There's just one problem: You have to get over the shock of turning chickpeas into cake! [Serves 8]

Vegetable oil spray

2 cups cooked chickpeas, drained (canned is okay)

6 egg whites or ½ cup + 1 tbsp. liquid egg white substitute

Zest of one lemon

Juice of one lemon (about ¼ cup)

1 tablespoon vanilla extract

1 cup brown Sugar Twin

½ cup granulated sugar

Directions

1. Preheat oven to 350 degrees F. Coat a pie dish with vegetable oil spray.

2. Combine chickpeas and egg whites in a food processor. Process until smooth.

3. Add lemon zest, lemon juice, vanilla, Sugar Twin, and sugar. Process again until smooth.

4. Transfer to pie dish and bake for 30–40 minutes, or until a knife inserted in the middle comes out clean.

5. Refrigerate leftovers.

Per Serving Calories: 138, Protein: 5 g, Carbohydrates: 27 g, Fiber: 3.1 g, Fat: 1.1 g, Saturated fat: 0.1 g, % of calories as fat: 7, Cholesterol: 0, Potassium: 152 mg, Sodium: 46 mg, Omega-3 fatty acids: 0

Exchanges Bread/starch: 0.7, Other carbs/sugar: 0.8, Very lean meat/protein: 0.5, Lean meat: 0, Fruit: 0, Vegetables: 0, Skim milk: 0, Fat: 0

FUDGEY BROWNIES

This recipe is perhaps one of my greatest pride and joys. I had to find a way to have chocolate healthfully. Making a black bean salad one day, the thought occurred to me that black beans and chocolate have something in common: their color. That was the start of my experimenting. The black beans lend both texture and substance, making up for the fat that has been removed. They also lend great fiber and minerals. The most important detail: These brownies are kid pleasing. [Serves 9]

Vegetable oil spray

½ cup cooked black beans (canned is okay)

⅓ cup liquid egg white substitute or 4 egg whites

½ cup granulated sugar

½ cup brown Sugar Twin

¼ cup canola-based, trans-fatty-acid-free margarine

½ cup all-purpose flour

2 ounces unsweetened Baker's chocolate, melted

2 tablespoons vanilla extract

Directions

1. Preheat oven to 350 degrees F. Coat a 9 × 9 pan with vegetable oil spray.

2. Place beans in a food processor with egg substitute and puree until smooth.

3. Transfer puree to a medium-size bowl. Add remaining ingredients and whisk together or use an electric mixer.

4. Transfer batter to pan and bake for 25 to 28 minutes. The batter should be slightly jiggly when removed from the oven.

Per Serving Calories: 178, Protein: 4 g, Carbohydrates: 21 g, Fiber: 2 g, Fat: 9 g, Saturated fat: 2.8 g, % of calories as fat: 43, Cholesterol: 0, Potassium: 144 mg, Sodium: 68 mg, Omega-3 fatty acids: 0

Exchanges Bread/starch: 0.5, Other carbs/sugar: 0.7, Very lean meat/protein: 0.2, Lean meat: 0, Fruit: 0, Vegetables: 0, Skim milk: 0, Fat: 1.7

TIRAMISU

I learned how to make the true Venetian version of Tiramisu while studying cooking in Venice. I then worked hard to make it a much healthier version. You won't even know you are eating something that is good for you! [Serves 5]

1 ounce Mascarpone cheese

4 ounces nonfat cream cheese

4 ounces nonfat sour cream

3 tablespoons granulated sugar

1 tablespoon Grand Marnier

2 tablespoons orange juice

Vegetable oil spray

4 ounces vanilla or lemon zest biscotti

¼ cup very strong coffee (add 1 tablespoon instant coffee to 6 ounces hot water)

¼ ounce dark chocolate bar, shaved

Directions

1. Bring the cheeses and sour cream to room temperature. Place them in a large bowl with the sugar and beat with an electric mixer or by hand until very smooth.

2. Beat in the Grand Marnier and orange juice.

3. Coat a springform pan with vegetable oil spray.

4. Dip biscotti, one at a time, in coffee briefly. Make a layer of these biscotti on the bottom. Spread half of cheese mixture evenly over the top.

5. Repeat, making another layer of biscotti and the cheese mixture on the top.

6. Place in the freezer, covered, for 1 hour or in refrigerator if not serving immediately. When ready to serve, sprinkle with shaved chocolate and then remove springform pan. Place on a pretty serving dish. Cut into 5 pieces.

Per Serving Calories: 221, Protein: 8 g, Carbohydrates: 27 g, Fiber: 0.8 g, Fat: 7.9 g, Saturated fat: 3.3 g, % of calories as fat: 32, Cholesterol: 15 mg, Potassium: 138 mg, Sodium: 228 mg, Omega-3 fatty acids: 0

Exchanges Bread/starch: 1.1, Other carbs/sugar: 0.4, Very lean meat/protein: 0.4, Lean meat: 0.1, Fruit: 0, Vegetables: 0, Skim milk: 0.2, Fat: 1.4

CHOCOLATE SILK MOUSSE

How many ways can you enjoy chocolate healthfully? Never enough, as far as I am concerned! [Serves 6]

½ cup water

2 packets unflavored gelatin

2 cups low-fat, fortified chocolate soy milk (preferably the Silk brand)

1½ cups fat-free Cool Whip or other frozen fat-free whipped topping

¼ cup light chocolate syrup

Directions

1. Heat water to boiling. Stir in gelatin and then continue to stir about 5 minutes or until gelatin is dissolved.

2. Pour chocolate milk into a large bowl. Whisk in gelatin mixture.

3. Whisk in Cool Whip and chocolate syrup.

4. Transfer mixture to 6 individual parfait glasses or to a bowl. Chill until set, 2 to 3 hours.

Per Serving Calories: 98, Protein: 6 g, Carbohydrates: 14 g, Fiber: 0.2 g, Fat: 1.4 g, Saturated fat: 0.2 g, % of calories as fat: 14, Cholesterol: 0, Potassium: 156 mg, Sodium: 66 mg, Omega-3 fatty acids: 0

Exchanges Bread/starch: 0.3, Other carbs/sugar: 0.7, Very lean meat/protein: 0.2, Lean meat: 0.4, Fruit: 0, Vegetables: 0, Skim milk: 0, Fat: 0

RASPBERRY CREAM GELATIN

Dessert doesn't have to be off limits—just well thought out. I had great fun in the kitchen developing this and the following gelatin recipes. My "don't-feed-me-healthy-food" family absolutely loves these desserts. This one is absolutely exquisite! [Serves 6]

One 16-ounce container fat-free cottage cheese
One 3-ounce package sugar-free raspberry gelatin
1½ cups boiling water
1 package Knox unflavored gelatin
3 cups fresh or frozen raspberries (no added sugar), thawed
2 cups fat-free Cool Whip

Directions

1. Puree cottage cheese in a food processor.

2. Blend raspberry gelatin with 1 cup boiling water, stirring well for about 3 minutes.

3. Blend unflavored gelatin with remaining ½ cup boiling water.

4. Place pureed cottage cheese and thawed raspberries in a large bowl and mix in Cool Whip.

5. Pour raspberry and unflavored gelatin mixtures over contents in bowl. Using a whisk, whip until smooth.

6. Place in a mold, 9 × 13 cake pan, or another appropriate container. Refrigerate until mixture has jelled, about 3 hours.

Per Serving (¾ cup) Calories: 175, Protein: 18 g, Carbohydrates: 23 g, Fiber: 4.2 g, Fat: 0.4 g, Saturated fat: 0, % of calories as fat: 2, Cholesterol: 6 mg, Potassium: 169 mg, Sodium: 592 mg, Omega-3 fatty acids: 0.1 g

Exchanges Bread/starch: 0, Other carbs/sugar: 1, Very lean meat/protein: 2.3, Lean meat: 0, Fruit: 0.5, Vegetables: 0, Skim milk: 0, Fat: 0

VANILLA PEACH MOUSSE

Just peachy, I say about this dessert. Whoever thought sneaking fruit into a dessert would have such fabulous results? [Serves 6]

Two 13-ounce cans peaches in water, drained
2 packages Knox unflavored gelatin
1 cup boiling water
12 ounces fat-free vanilla yogurt (100 calories per 6 ounces)

Directions

1. Puree peaches in a food processor or blender.

2. Blend both packages of unflavored gelatin into boiling water, stirring well for about 3 minutes.

3. Place pureed peaches and yogurt into a mixing bowl. Pour dissolved gelatin over the top and whisk until mixture is uniformly smooth and creamy.

4. Transfer to 6 parfait glasses or a covered, flat container and refrigerate 3 to 4 hours, or until mixture has jelled.

Per Serving (¾ cup) Calories: 74, Protein: 5 g, Carbohydrates: 13 g, Fiber: 1.6 g, Fat: 0.1 g, Saturated fat: 0, % of calories as fat: 1, Cholesterol: 2 mg, Potassium: 121 mg, Sodium: 51 mg, Omega-3 fatty acids: 0

Exchanges Bread/starch: 0, Other carbs/sugar: 0, Very lean meat/protein: 0.2, Lean meat: 0, Fruit: 0.5, Vegetables: 0, Skim milk: 0.4, Fat: 0

APRICOT CREAM

Gentle and yet bold, this fabulous dessert will become a favorite. [Serves 6]

Two 15-ounce cans apricots in water
One 16-ounce container fat-free cottage cheese
One 3-ounce package sugar-free orange gelatin
1 cup boiling water

Directions

1. Drain apricots and puree with cottage cheese in a food processor or blender.

2. In a bowl, pour boiling water into gelatin powder, stirring until well dissolved.

3. Place pureed apricots and vanilla yogurt into mixing bowl.

4. Pour dissolved gelatin over the top.

5. Whisk well until mixture is uniformly smooth and creamy.

6. Cover and refrigerate about 3 to 4 hours, or until mixture has jelled.

Per Serving (about ¾ cup) Calories: 88, Protein: 11 g, Carbohydrates: 12 g, Fiber: 2.3 g, Fat: 0.2 g, Saturated fat: 0, % of calories as fat: 2, Cholesterol: 6 mg, Potassium: 321 mg, Sodium: 234 mg, Omega-3 fatty acids: 0

Exchanges Bread/starch: 0, Other carbs/sugar: 0, Very lean meat/protein: 1.3, Lean meat: 0, Fruit: 0.6, Vegetables: 0, Skim milk: 0, Fat: 0

TRAIL MIX

Enjoy dried fruit and nuts in a combination that works for your taste buds and your health. [Serves 1]

2 tablespoons dried cranberries
2 tablespoons almonds
2 tablespoons raisins

Directions

Mix all ingredients together and enjoy.

Per Serving Calories: 202, Protein: 4 g, Carbohydrates: 28 g, Fiber: 2.1 g, Fat: 10.1 g, Saturated fat: 0.8 g, % of calories as fat: 42, Cholesterol: 0, Potassium: 275 mg, Sodium: 6 mg, Omega-3 fatty acids: 0

Exchanges Bread/starch: 0, Other carbs/sugar: 0, Very lean meat/protein: 0.4, Lean meat: 0, Fruit: 1.6, Vegetables: 0, Skim milk: 0, Fat: 2

Side Dishes

HERBED RED-SKINNED POTATOES

Who doesn't love French fries? Here's a great alternative that will soon be your preference. I love to make this with tiny new potatoes when they're available. [Serves 4]

1 pound red potatoes
2 tablespoons extra-virgin olive oil
1 tablespoon Mrs. Dash Classic Italiano or Italian seasoning

Directions

1. Preheat oven to 350 degrees F. Coat a baking sheet with vegetable oil spray.

2. Scrub potatoes and cut into large bite-size pieces, leaving peel on as many slices as possible.

3. Brush with oil and sprinkle with Mrs. Dash seasoning.

4. Bake for 20 minutes, turning once after 10 minutes.

Per Serving Calories: 187, Protein: 3 g, Carbohydrates: 29 g, Fiber: 2.7 g, Fat: 7.1 g, Saturated fat: 1 g, % of calories as fat: 34, Cholesterol: 0, Potassium: 474 mg, Sodium: 9.1 mg, Omega-3 fatty acids: 0.1 g

Exchanges Bread/starch: 1.7, Other carbs/sugar: 0, Very lean meat/protein: 0, Lean meat: 0, Fruit: 0, Vegetables: 0, Skim milk: 0, Fat: 1.4

TOMATO-BASIL RICE PILAF

This wonderfully colorful, texture-rich, and truly delicious rice is so quick and easy to make that you'll enjoy it yourself. It's so gourmet-tasting that you can serve it for guests. It is especially great with grilled chicken or fish. [Serves 2]

2 teaspoons canola oil
½ cup chopped green onions
½ cup instant brown rice
⅔ cup water

1 cup chopped sun-dried tomatoes
2 teaspoons Mrs. Dash Tomato-Basil Garlic or
 ½ teaspoon dried basil
½ cup frozen peas

Directions

1. In a medium nonstick skillet, heat oil over medium heat.

2. Add onions and sauté until slightly browned and wilted.

3. Add rice, water, tomatoes, and Mrs. Dash seasoning. Stir, cover, and simmer for 10 minutes.

4. Add peas and simmer just to heat peas through, about 5 minutes.

Per Serving Calories: 200, Protein: 7 g, Carbohydrates: 33 g, Fiber: 6.5 g, Fat: 5.9 g, Saturated fat: 0.6 g, % of calories as fat: 25, Cholesterol: 0, Potassium: 1,086 mg, Sodium: 614 mg, Omega-3 fatty acids: 0.4 g

Exchanges Bread/starch: 1, Other carbs/sugar: 0, Very lean meat/protein: 0, Lean meat: 0, Fruit: 0, Vegetables: 3.2, Skim milk: 0, Fat: 0.9

ORANGE BULGUR PILAF

Using orange juice to perk up bulgur creates an interesting flavor. Use this cold as the basis for a salad. Or use it hot, under fish, tofu stir-fries, or grilled chicken. [Serves 6]

1½ cups uncooked bulgur
¾ cup boiling water
4 teaspoons extra-virgin olive oil
¾ cup fresh orange juice

¼ teaspoon salt
¼ teaspoon black pepper
½ cup chopped fresh parsley
10 large black olives, pitted and chopped

Directions

1. Place bulgur in a small bowl and pour boiling water over it. Add oil and stir for a few minutes, allowing the bulgur to open up.

2. Stir in the orange juice, salt, pepper, and parsley. Cover tightly and let stand at room temperature for 30 minutes, stirring occasionally.

3. Stir in the olives.

Per Serving Calories: 178, Protein: 5 g, Carbohydrates: 31 g, Fiber: 6.7 g, Fat: 5.1 g, Saturated fat: 0.5 g, % of calories as fat: 24, Cholesterol: 0, Potassium: 234 mg, Sodium: 167 mg, Omega-3 fatty acids: 0.03 g

Exchanges Bread/starch: 1.5, Other carbs/sugar: 0, Very lean meat/protein: 0, Lean meat: 0, Fruit: 0.2, Vegetables: 0.1, Skim milk: 0, Fat: 0.7

CREAMY ROASTED RED PEPPER AND LENTIL DIP

Who said dips have to be unhealthy? I've created a great one that is loaded with fiber as well as antioxidants. It can be stored in the refrigerator for several days. Served at a party, this is sure to be a hit—even if you aren't a fan of lentils. [Serves 1]

1 cup uncooked lentils
2 green tea bags
1 cup roasted red peppers (about one 7.25-ounce jar, in water or brine, not oil, drained)
⅓ cup fat-free sour cream

Directions

1. Cook lentils with 2 tea bags and 3 cups water for 45 minutes, or until lentils are tender.

2. Puree lentils, red peppers, and sour cream in a food processor. Use for dipping veggies and crackers or for spreading on whole grain bread for a sandwich.

Per Serving Calories: 373, Protein: 25 g, Carbohydrates: 64 g, Fiber: 17 g, Fat: 3.1 g, Saturated fat: 1.1 g, % of calories as fat: 7, Cholesterol: 8 mg, Potassium: 918 mg, Sodium: 814 mg, Omega-3 fatty acids: 0.07 g

Exchanges Bread/starch: 2.6, Other carbs/sugar: 0, Very lean meat/protein: 0.4, Lean meat: 0, Fruit: 0, Vegetables: 2.3, Skim milk: 0.8, Fat: 0.5

BACON-CHEDDAR POTATO SKINS

Part of the fun and the wonder of learning about healthy eating is that you learn to retool your cooking repertoire so that you can enjoy something like these potato skins. You will absolutely love them. Serve them as dinner, as a snack, or at your next party. The vegetable bacon is often called vegetable breakfast strips and can be found in the freezer case. If you cannot find them, substitute Canadian bacon, found in the meat case. [Serves 4]

2 large baking potatoes
Vegetable oil spray
6 slices vegetable bacon
½ cup chopped green onions
⅓ cup cooked black beans (canned is okay, but drain before measuring)
½ teaspoon cumin

½ teaspoon chili powder
2 tablespoons water
1 teaspoon canola oil
4 ounces 50% fat-reduced cheddar cheese, grated
Jalapeño peppers to taste, chopped (optional)
½ cup fat-free sour cream

Directions

1. Preheat oven to 350 degrees F. Coat a cookie sheet with vegetable oil spray.

2. Scrub the potatoes and pierce with a fork. Place in oven and bake until fork-tender, 45 to 60 minutes.

3. Place bacon on the cookie sheet in 1 layer. Place in oven with potatoes and cook according to package instructions until crisp. Remove from oven and allow to cool. (The bacon will be done in 12 to 15 minutes, much sooner than the potatoes.)

4. Remove potatoes from oven and cut in half lengthwise. Set aside to cool.

5. Coat a medium-size nonstick skillet with vegetable oil spray and heat over medium-high heat.

6. Add onions, black beans, cumin, chili powder, and water. Cook, stirring constantly, until water has evaporated.

7. Remove pan from heat and place mixture in a bowl. Add bacon to bowl, crumbling it into tiny pieces. Mix well. Do not wash pan because leftover spices will flavor potato skins in the next step.

8. Scoop about half of flesh from potato skins.

9. Place one-fourth of bacon mixture in each potato skin.

(continued)

10. Sprinkle one-fourth of cheese (about ¼ cup) on top of filled potato skin.

11. Add oil to pan in which you sautéed onion and black beans. Heat over medium heat.

12. Place filled potato skins in hot oil, leaning against each other.

13. Sprinkle remaining cheese evenly over potato skins. Add jalapeño peppers if desired.

14. Cover and cook 10 to 15 minutes, or until cheese has melted.

15. Serve each portion with 2 tablespoons sour cream.

Per Serving Calories: 243, Protein: 14 g, Carbohydrates: 27 g, Fiber: 3.7 g, Fat: 9.7 g, Saturated fat: 3.9 g, % of calories as fat: 35, Cholesterol: 18 mg, Potassium: 378 mg, Sodium: 436 mg, Omega-3 fatty acids: 0.11 g

Exchanges Bread/starch: 1.2, Other carbs/sugar: 0, Very lean meat/protein: 0.1, Lean meat: 1.3, Fruit: 0, Vegetables: 0.3, Skim milk: 0.3, Fat: 1.1

CARAMELIZED ONION AND PARMESAN BRUSCHETTA

A bruschetta you can eat every day! This one is piled high with vitamin- and phyto-chemical-rich vegetables, and just the right amount of regular cheese. This recipe demonstrates that you can have regular cheese if you learn to augment it with healthier versions such as soy cheese and nonfat versions. [Serves 16]

1 tablespoon extra-virgin olive oil

2 red onions, peeled, thinly sliced, and separated into rings

½ teaspoon black pepper

1 tablespoon packed brown sugar

One 16-ounce loaf fat-free ciabatta, Italian, or French bread

One 12-ounce jar Walden Farms Bruschetta sauce

8 ounces mushrooms, sliced

Eight ⅔ -ounce slices mozzarella-flavored soy cheese

2 ounces Parmesan cheese (regular fat), shredded

4 ounces fat-free Parmesan cheese, shredded

1 ripe tomato, very thinly sliced

½ cup freshly chopped parsley

Directions

1. Heat oil in a nonstick skillet over medium-low heat. Add onions, pepper, and sugar. Turn occasionally but allow onions to brown before turning. Cook until wilted and delicately browned.

2. Preheat oven to 400 degrees F.

3. Cut bread in half lengthwise. Line 2 cookie sheets with aluminum foil and place one half on each cookie sheet.

4. Spread half of the bruschetta on each loaf half, using a rubber spatula to cover the entire surface.

5. Sprinkle mushrooms evenly over bread.

6. Spread caramelized onions evenly over the mushrooms.

7. Place 4 slices soy cheese on each half, distributing evenly.

8. In a small bowl, mix Parmesan cheeses. Sprinkle evenly over both halves. Top with tomato slices.

9. Bake about 15 minutes, or until the bread is crispy on the bottom and the cheese begins to bubble.

10. Remove from oven and garnish with parsley. Cut each half into 8 slices.

Per Serving Calories: 171, Protein: 9 g, Carbohydrates: 18 g, Fiber: 1.3 g, Fat: 6.3 g, Saturated fat: 1.1 g, % of calories as fat: 34, Cholesterol: 4.1 mg, Potassium: 129 mg, Sodium: 465 mg, Omega-3 fatty acids: 0.02 g

Exchanges Bread/starch: 1, Other carbs/sugar: 0, Very lean meat/protein: 0.3, Lean meat: 0.2, Fruit: 0, Vegetables: 0.4, Skim milk: 0, Fat: 0.3

THAT'S A CHEESY NACHO

Whoever said you cannot have cheesy nachos again? Try this version, and you'll be in love! [Serves 4]

1 tablespoon fresh or bottled lime juice
½ teaspoon chili powder
½ teaspoon ground cumin
½ teaspoon garlic powder
½ teaspoon cayenne pepper
6 corn taco shells
Vegetable oil spray

4 ounces 50% reduced-fat cheddar cheese, grated
Jalapeño peppers to taste, chopped (optional)
2 tomatoes, chopped
½ cup chopped green onions
½ cup minced fresh cilantro
½ cup fat-free sour cream

Directions

1. Preheat oven to 400 degrees F.

2. In a small bowl, mix lime juice, chili powder, cumin, garlic powder, and cayenne pepper. The mixture will be very thick.

3. Break taco shells in half.

4. Coat a cookie sheet with vegetable oil spray.

5. Spread each side of shell with a thin layer of lime juice-spice mixture and place shells on cookie sheet.

6. Place in preheated oven for 1 minute, just to set spices.

7. Spread cheese evenly over shells. Top with jalapeño peppers if desired.

8. Return shells to oven.

9. Bake for 2 to 4 minutes, just until cheese melts.

10. Serve with sides of chopped tomatoes, green onions, cilantro, and sour cream.

Per Serving Calories: 212, Protein: 12 g, Carbohydrates: 25 g, Fiber: 3 g, Fat: 9.1 g, Saturated fat: 4.1 g, % of calories as fat: 36, Cholesterol: 18 mg, Potassium: 270 mg, Sodium: 350 mg, Omega-3 fatty acids: 0.01 g

Exchanges Bread/starch: 0, Other carbs/sugar: 0, Very lean meat/protein: 0, Lean meat: 1.1, Fruit: 0, Vegetables: 0.8, Skim milk: 0.3, Fat: 0.3

ZESTY CAULIFLOWER SALAD

Looking for an easy vegetable or a dish to take to a picnic? This is the one you're looking for. The color is inviting, and the flavor is spectacular. [Serves 4]

1 pound frozen cauliflower, thawed
½ cup frozen petite peas, thawed
One 7.25-ounce jar roasted red peppers, drained and chopped
¼ cup light Miracle Whip (preferably) or reduced-fat mayonnaise

1–3 teaspoons horseradish (depending on how much zip you like)
1 tablespoon lemon juice
¼ teaspoon salt
Ground black pepper to taste

Directions

1. Place cauliflower, peas, and red peppers in a medium-size bowl.

2. In a small bowl, whisk together Miracle Whip, horseradish, lemon juice, salt, and pepper. Pour over vegetables and use a rubber spatula to coat all of them.

Per Serving Calories: 98, Protein: 4 g, Carbohydrates: 13 g, Fiber: 3.8 g, Fat: 3.9 g, Saturated fat: 0.8 g, % of calories as fat: 34, Cholesterol: 5 mg, Potassium: 255 mg, Sodium: 513 mg, Omega-3 fatty acids: 0.1 g

Exchanges Bread/starch: 0.2, Other carbs/sugar: 0.2, Very lean meat/protein: 0, Lean meat: 0, Fruit: 0, Vegetables: 1.7, Skim milk: 0, Fat: 0.7

HEARTY MULTIGRAIN BREAD

I have found that my Kitchen-Aid mixer makes baking homemade bread a snap. I start with the wire whip and then switch to the dough hook as I proceed. I consider the mixer an investment in my health. This recipe makes four loaves, twelve slices each. You can freeze the leftovers. [Serves 48]

2 cups dry oat bran
2 cups milled or ground flaxseed
2 cups toasted wheat germ
1 tablespoon salt, Kosher salt, or sea salt

1 cup boiling water
¼ cup extra-virgin olive oil
¼ cup molasses
½ cup warm water
3 tablespoons (cakes) yeast

¼ cup packed brown sugar
½ cup vital wheat gluten
3 cups all-purpose flour
Vegetable oil spray

Directions

1. In a large mixing bowl, combine oat bran, flaxseed, wheat germ, salt, and boiling water. Stir by hand or mix with a wire whisk on an electric mixer.

2. Whisk in oil and molasses. Let sit as you prepare the yeast.

3. In a small bowl, whisk together warm but not hot water, yeast, and sugar. Set aside.

4. Blend vital wheat gluten into oat bran mixture by hand or with a wire whisk on mixer.

5. Use a rubber spatula to scrape the yeast mixture into the oat bran mixture. Stir vigorously by hand or with a wire whisk for 3 minutes.

6. Add 1 cup flour. Blend with a spoon or with a wire whisk on mixer.

7. If using a mixer, change to dough hook and add remaining flour, 1 cup at a time. If using dough hook, knead 3 to 5 minutes. Knead by hand about the same amount of time.

8. Coat 4 large loaf pans with vegetable oil spray.

9. Divide dough into 4 equal balls. Shape into loaves and transfer to loaf pans. Cover to prevent air drafts from reaching loaves and let rise until double in size, about 1 hour.

10. About 45 minutes after setting bread to rise, preheat oven to 350 degrees F. Bake 35 to 45 minutes, or until lightly golden brown.

Per Serving (1 slice) Calories: 119, Protein: 5 g, Carbohydrates: 16 g, Fiber: 2.5 g, Fat: 4.2 g, Saturated fat: 0.3 g, % of calories as fat: 31, Cholesterol: 0, Potassium: 137 mg, Sodium: 147 mg, Omega-3 fatty acids: 0.1 g

Exchanges Bread/starch: 0.8, Other carbs/sugar: 0.1, Very lean meat/protein: 0.2, Lean meat: 0.2, Fruit: 0, Vegetables: 0, Skim milk: 0, Fat: 0.6

KRIS'S HIGHEST FIBER (AND MOISTEST) BREAD

Turn your bread into a celebration of health. This bread is so fabulous, you'll think you're having dessert. When I make a loaf, I slice it and freeze the slices so that it always has a just-baked fresh taste. This recipe makes four loaves, twelve slices each. Make a batch and freeze the rest. [Serves 48]

2 cups cooked lentils
3 cups oat bran
2 cups ground flaxseed
1 cup wheat germ
1 tablespoon salt
¼ cup olive oil

¼ cup molasses
½ cup warm water
3 tablespoons (cakes) yeast
¼ cup packed brown sugar
½ cup vital wheat gluten
4 cups all-purpose flour

Directions

1. In a large mixing bowl, combine lentils, oat bran, flaxseed, wheat germ, salt, oil, and molasses. Stir by hand or mix with a wire whisk on an electric mixer.

2. In a small bowl, whisk together warm but not hot water, yeast, and sugar. Set aside.

3. Blend vital wheat gluten into lentil mixture by hand or with a wire whisk on mixer.

4. Use a rubber spatula to scrape the yeast mixture into the lentil mixture. Stir vigorously by hand or with a wire whisk for 3 minutes.

5. Add 1 cup flour. Blend with a spoon or with a wire whisk on mixer.

6. If using a mixer, change to dough hook and add remaining flour, 1 cup at a time. If using dough hook, knead 3 to 5 minutes. Knead by hand about the same amount of time.

7. Coat 4 large loaf pans with vegetable oil spray.

8. Divide dough into 4 equal balls. Shape into loaves and transfer to loaf pans. Cover to prevent air drafts from reaching loaves and let rise until double in size, about 1 hour.

9. About 45 minutes after setting bread to rise, preheat oven to 350 degrees F. Bake 35 to 45 minutes, or until lightly golden brown.

Per Serving Calories: 130, Protein: 5 g, Carbohydrates: 19 g, Fiber: 2.6 g, Fat: 4.1 g, Saturated fat: 0.3 g, % of calories as fat: 27, Cholesterol: 0, Potassium: 131 mg, Sodium: 148 mg, Omega-3 fatty acids: 1 g

Exchanges Bread/starch: 1, Other carbs/sugar: 0.2, Very lean meat/protein: 0, Lean meat: 0.2, Fruit: 0, Vegetables: 0, Skim milk: 0, Fat: 0.6

Index